Quick and Easy
Wall Pilates Workouts
to Transform Your Body in 28 Days

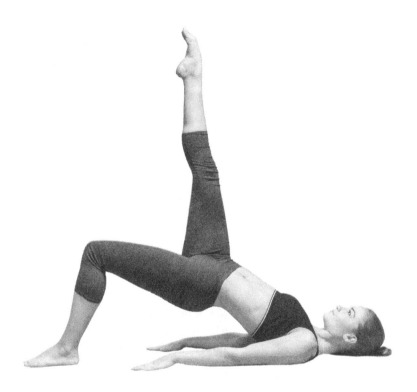

The complete challenge will **sculpt the body in 28 days**, toning buttocks, legs, belly and arms
with illustrated exercises for the whole body.

Just 15 minutes of targeted training per day is all it takes to slim down and regain muscle tone, flexibility and strength.

Rachel White

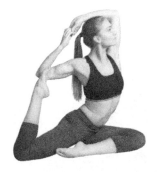

This book is dedicated to all the women who want to take care of themselves while respecting their daily rhythms and cycles.

Rachel White

BONUS: *Progress Journal*

Welcome to this new adventure! To successfully complete the challenge you are about to begin, I recommend that you use the self-assessment progress journal which I have created for you. This journal is meant to motivate you along the way, because the hardest part of any new project is not starting it, but completing it.

How many times have you begun a diet and then abandoned it? How many times have you thought about joining a gym and then didn't? This is your unique opportunity to change that! Through the self-assessment method, it will be easier to reach your goal because the results you get day by day will motivate you to continue.

Why is it important to finish the challenge? Because by reaching the end of the 28 days, you will be able to see your physique transformed, plus you will have internalized a new daily routine that will keep you fit for months and years to come!

Download the journal using this link:
https://wallpilatestotalbody.flyedition.com/
or scan the QR code!

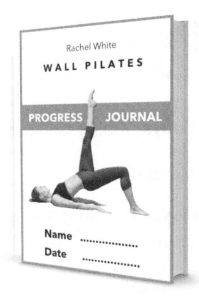

The progress journal will help you to:

- Set realistic goals
- Track the changes in your body
- Monitor other benefits such as increased physical strength, straighter posture, improved flexibility, and better balance and coordination.

SUMMARY

Introduction

Benefits of Wall Pilates

I am thrilled to hear that you are about to begin this new challenge, and I hope that my book will give you a life-changing experience! Perhaps you, like me, initially chose Wall Pilates because you were looking for a way to lose weight and firm the body that was easy and could be done at home. Aesthetic goals, in fact, are normally what drives a person to start a physical activity but, trust me, Wall Pilates is not just a muscle workout for a more toned shape!

Wall Pilates is a complete workout that will make you more beautiful and confident!

- Wall Pilates has many benefits that need to be taken into consideration and that have motivated me to continue practicing it for many years. That is why with this book I want to give you the best possible experience and guide you step by step in the correct execution of the exercises, to help you get the most out of your workouts. Read carefully about all the benefits you can get, so that you can increase your awareness of the path you are beginning and fully understand the goals you want to achieve. The self-assessment form you downloaded will help you track these goals.

- Increased strength: Pilates is known to increase the strength of all the muscles in the body, and Pilates at the wall is no exception! With consistent training you will feel more confident in performing daily activities such as climbing stairs, grocery shopping, mowing the lawn, cleaning the house, and carrying heavy bags. Life will feel lighter and easier to you.

- Improved posture: Wall Pilates provides a stable surface to support your body during your workout. This helps you to have greater awareness of your body position and to maintain proper alignment during exercises, resulting in reduced neck, shoulder, back, and hip pain.

- Increased flexibility: Wall Pilates incorporates stretching and flexibility exercises that help increase your elasticity. Picking up objects on the floor, getting dressed and tying your shoes will be activities you can do with much greater ease.

- Improved balance and coordination: Pilates exercises at the Wall involve training in leg and arm coordination and require stability when performing the exercises. This is especially beneficial for people recovering from injuries and helps with concentration and coordination.

- Gentle on joints: If you haven't exercised for a long time or if you have noticed pain in your hips and knees from doing strenuous exercise, Wall Pilates is the best possible option because the wall provides support and reduces the impact on your joints without limiting your ability to strengthen your muscles and firm your body.

- Finally, Wall Pilates strengthens women's pelvic floor: A weak pelvic floor can lead to unintentional urine leakage during physical activity or when coughing or lifting heavy objects. Wall Pilates prevents and resolves urinary incontinence, particularly after pregnancy and childbirth or due to tissue relaxation due to aging. In addition, the pelvic floor provides support to internal organs such as the bladder, uterus, and rectum, so strengthening the pelvic floor helps prevent prolapse and maintains the overall health of your genital system.

Wall Pilates is also a workout for the mind, not just the body! Stay focused on the movements and breathing to enhance the benefits of the practice!

Learning the Correct Position

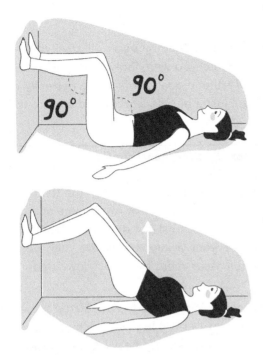

To get started, you need to follow some technical tips so that you can perform a safe and effective workout. Choose the right distance from the wall to perform the "bridge position". Your feet should be at knee height so that they form a 90-degree angle. Your knees in turn should form a 90-degree angle with your hip joints, so you need to make sure your hips are just below your knees. This way you can get into the "bridge" position and achieve full hip extension, using your glutes to push up.

Be careful: If you feel too much pressure in the hamstrings, you may have to lower or raise your feet and may have to move closer to or away from the wall. Find your ideal position especially at first, with the ambition of being able to achieve the perfect position later, so you can avoid putting too much effort into it. The position to hold during the first few weeks of training is the one that gives you the feeling that you can actually push against the wall, to get the maximum possible hip extension.

If during the exercises you feel the need to move and position yourself closer to the wall, that is perfectly fine; the important thing is that throughout the workout you are pain-free. The exercises may make you struggle but they should not cause you pain; if they do, it likely means you are in the wrong position.

When you perform the exercises, take breaks. Breaks may seem unnecessary, but they are important to enable you to complete the whole workout at a steady pace, rather than starting very fast and stopping in the middle because you're in pain and feel tired.

Note that some exercises are repeated, with the difference being only the speed – once slowly or following your natural breathing pattern, and once with more speed. They should feel different when performed slowly versus dynamically, so take note of how your body responds to each set.

What You Need to Get Started

- An important aspect of a successful challenge is to know in advance what you need to make it as easy as possible to get going, so that there are no obstacles or problems to interrupt you. As the days go by, the initial enthusiasm may wane and everyday commitments may distract you from your goals, so it is important to follow these simple tips.

- Avoid doing your exercises in a different place each day and having to move furniture or rugs or take pictures off the wall: The easier it is to access your workout area, the easier it will be to complete your 28-day challenge. Having to tidy up the room after your workout is an extra chore which may make you decide to skip some workouts.

- Choose a location in the house where there is enough room to rest your feet on the wall and move your arms freely. Make sure there are no obstacles (pictures, radiators, furniture or anything else) or objects that could fall on you and injure you.

- Use a soft, non-slip mat on which to lie so that you can maintain the correct position during the exercises. You will thus avoid slipping and having to constantly reposition yourself.

- Choose a time of day when you will have no distractions and turn off your cell phone. Remember that Wall Pilates is also a workout for the mind, not just the body. It is important to stay focused on the movements and breathing to enhance the benefits of the practice.

- Wear comfortable clothing and avoid hairstyles that do not allow you to rest your head flat on the floor. Use a pillow to do the final relaxation or perform the exercises on your knees.

Make Your Own Equipment at Home

Some of the proposed exercises require the use of tools to intensify the workout. If you own these tools, you can use them; otherwise I suggest you make them at home. This way you will have no additional costs.

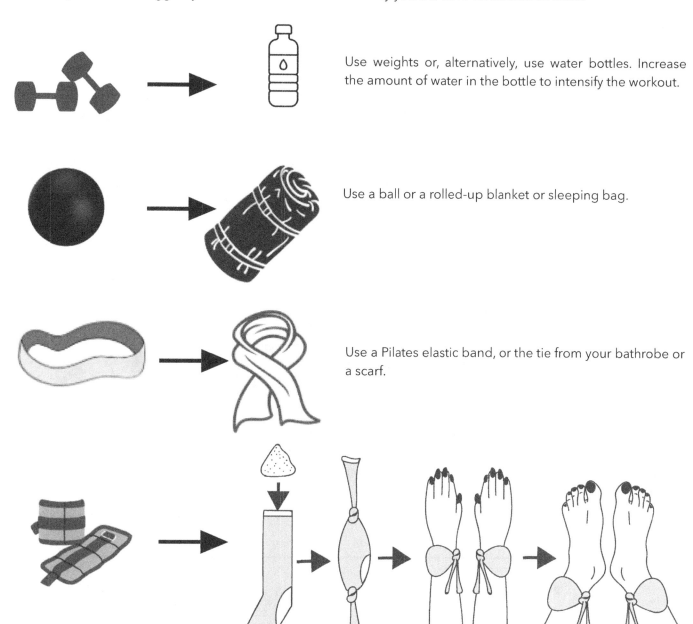

Use weights or, alternatively, use water bottles. Increase the amount of water in the bottle to intensify the workout.

Use a ball or a rolled-up blanket or sleeping bag.

Use a Pilates elastic band, or the tie from your bathrobe or a scarf.

Use ankle and wrist weights or fill a sock with sand and tie knots at both ends. Increase the amount of sand in the sock to intensify the workout.

You're ready to get started!

WORKOUT DAY 1

Exercise 1

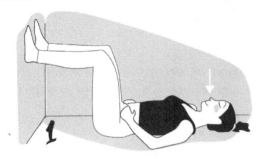 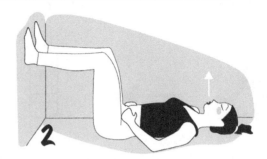

1. Rest your feet on the wall and rest your hands on your belly. Keep your eyes closed. Breathe in slowly through your nose until you feel your belly rise under your hands.

2. Exhale slowly with your mouth ajar, relaxing the muscles in your face. Repeat for 2 minutes.

Exercise 2

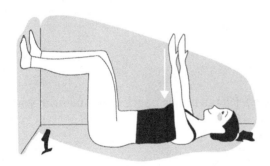 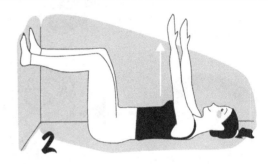

1. Keep your gaze upward and your feet firm against the wall. Maintain slow breathing and relaxed facial muscles. Bring arms outstretched overhead with shoulders firmly on the floor and palms facing inward.

2. Stretch your arms upward by pulling your shoulders off the ground, without arching your back, then return with your shoulders resting on the ground.

Perform the movement dynamically (briskly, with energy) 15 times, then pause for 15 seconds. Repeat 3 times.

Exercise 3

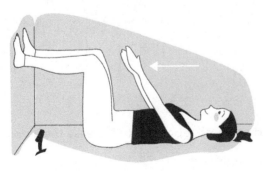 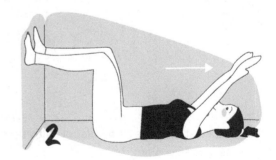

1.Keep your gaze upward and your feet firm against the wall. Exhale and bring your outstretched arms toward your knees without arching your back and contract your abdominals.

2.Inhale and bring your outstretched arms back past your gaze.

Perform the movement following the breath 15 times, then pause for 15 seconds. Repeat 3 times.

Exercise 4

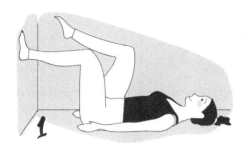 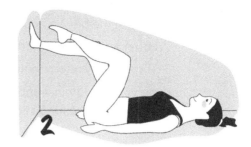

1.Keep your gaze upward. Exhale and bring your right knee toward your chest as you contract your abs.

2.Inhale and bring your foot back against the wall. Exhale and bring your left knee toward your chest as you contract your abs. Inhale and bring your foot back against the wall.

Perform the movements following the breath 15 times, then pause for 15 seconds. Repeat 3 times.

Exercise 5

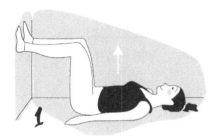 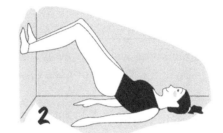 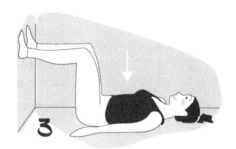

1. Keep your gaze upward. Inhale and slowly lift your pelvis up to the bridge position, making sure to raise one vertebra at a time off the floor until you bring your weight onto your shoulder blades.

2. Look upward in a way that promotes breathing. Hold the position for a few seconds.

3. Exhale and slowly roll your back towards the floor, letting one vertebra rest at a time, to return to the starting position.

Perform the movement slowly, following the rhythm of your breath, 15 times, then pause for 15 seconds before doing the next exercise.

Exercise 6

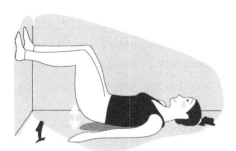 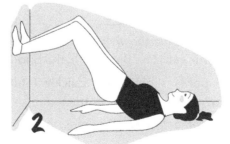 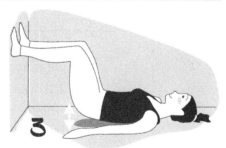

1. Keep your gaze upward, your feet firm against the wall, and your pelvis slightly raised off the ground.

2. Inhale and slowly lift your pelvis to a bridge position. Hold the position for a few seconds.

3. Exhale and return to the starting position with the pelvis slightly lifted off the ground.

Perform the movement slowly, following the rhythm of your breath, 15 times, then pause for 15 seconds before doing the next exercise.

Exercise 7

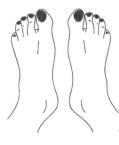

1. Keep your feet close together and firm against the wall with your pelvis lifted off the ground in the bridge position. Keep your gaze upward.

2. Lower your pelvis slightly.

3. Then quickly return to the bridge position.

Keep your abdominal and gluteal muscles contracted. Perform the movement quickly 20 times, then pause for 5 seconds. Repeat 3 times.

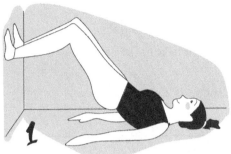 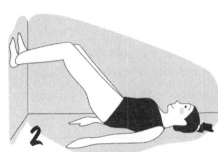 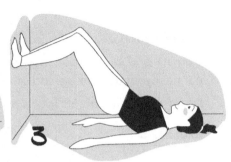

Exercise 8

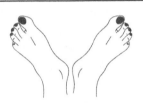

1. Rest your feet against the wall, toes away from each other, and lift your pelvis off the floor in the bridge position. Keep your gaze upward.

2. Lower the pelvis slightly.

3. Then quickly return to the bridge position. Keep your abdominal and gluteal muscles contracted.

Perform the movement quickly 20 times, then pause for 5 seconds. Repeat 3 times.

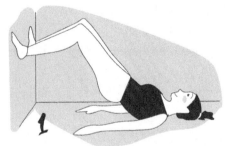 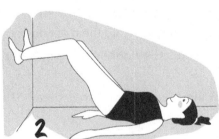 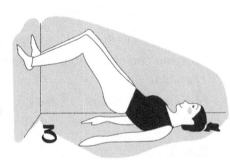

Exercise 9

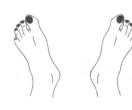

1. Rest your feet against the wall, spaced apart, with your toes pointed away from each other, and lift your pelvis off the floor in the bridge position. Keep your gaze upward.

2. Lower the pelvis slightly and quickly return to the bridge position. Keep your abdominal and gluteal muscles contracted.

Perform the movement quickly 15 times, then pause for 15 seconds. Repeat 3 times

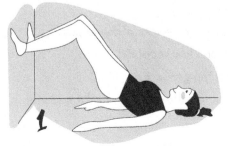 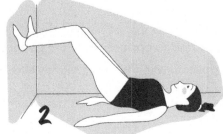 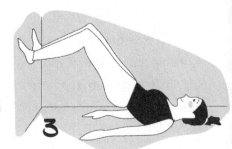

Exercise 10

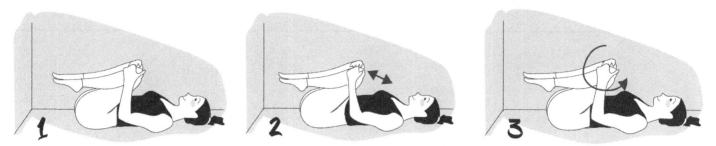

1. Bring your knees against your chest and put your hands on your knees. Take long breaths for 1 minute.

2. Then bring your knees closer to and away from your chest in a gentle motion for 1 minute.

3. Finally, make rotating movements with your knees to the right and left for 1 minute. This is a gentle massage for your back.

Final relaxation

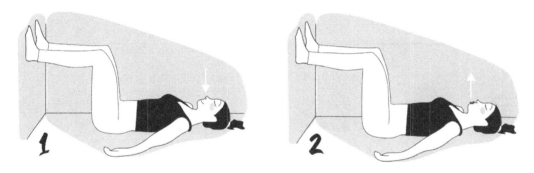

1. Rest your feet on the wall and keep your arms along your sides. Breathe in slowly through your nose. Keep your eyes closed.

2. Exhale slowly with your mouth ajar and relax your body muscles. Repeat for 1 minute.

Tip of the Day: Alternative breakfast ideas

My favorite meal? Breakfast! For years I had been searching for the right compromise between lightness and energy, and I finally found it. A large cup of kukicha, which is a naturally caffeine-free Japanese tea. One tablespoon of honey. Five almonds and one walnut. Three fat-free, dairy-free cookies. One piece of fruit.

And have you found your ideal breakfast? Choose from healthy ingredients such as toast, jam, yogurt, oat milk and many other alternatives you can find in the supermarket and limit your use of caffeine, fat and sugar.

Every person is different, and each person must find his or her perfect balance between energy and lightness.

WORKOUT DAY 2

Exercise 1

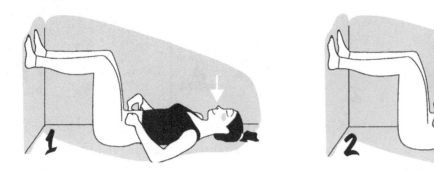

1. Rest your feet on the wall and keep your hands on your hips. Keep your eyes closed. Breathe in slowly through your nose and rotate your pelvis forward slightly (keep your lumbar vertebrae on the floor).

2. Exhale slowly with your mouth ajar and rotate your pelvis back slightly (keep your lumbar vertebrae off the floor). Repeat for 2 minutes.

Exercise 2

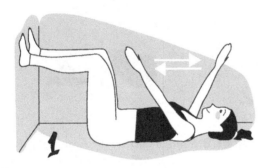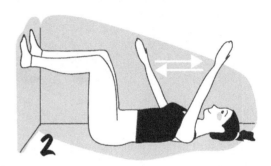

1. Keep your gaze upward and your feet firm against the wall. Bring your outstretched arms up with your shoulders resting firmly on the floor.

2. Perform an energetic movement by alternating your arms forward and backward.

Perform the movement 15 times, then pause for 15 seconds. Repeat 3 times.

Exercise 3

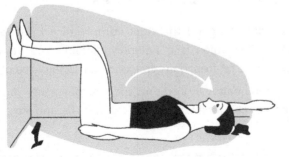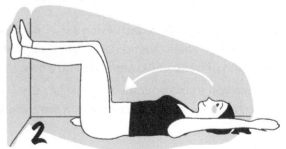

1. Keep your gaze upward and your feet firm against the wall. Exhale and place your arms by your sides, one up and one down, and contract your abs.

2. Inhale and alternate the position of the arms slowly, following your breath.

Perform the movement in rhythm with your breath 15 times, then pause for 15 seconds. Repeat 3 times.

Exercise 4

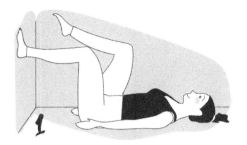 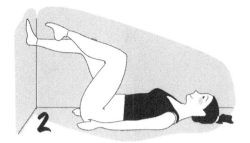

1. Keep your gaze upward. Bring your right knee toward your chest as you contract your abs.

2. Place your foot back against the wall and bring your left knee toward your chest as you contract your abs.

Perform the movements dynamically (briskly, with energy) 15 times, then pause for 15 seconds. Repeat 3 times.

Exercise 5

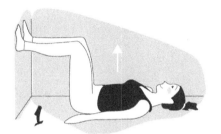 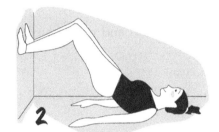 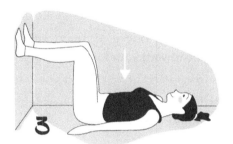

1. Keep your back on the floor, feet resting on the wall and look upward.

2. Lift your pelvis to the bridge position. Contract your glutes.

3. Return to the starting position with your pelvis on the floor and repeat.

Perform the movement dynamically 15 times, then pause for 15 seconds before doing the next exercise.

Exercise 6

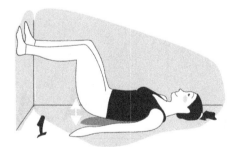 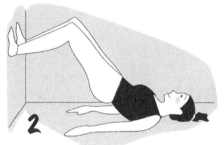 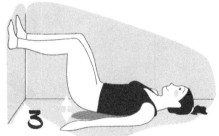

1. Keep the pelvis slightly raised off the ground.

2. Raise the pelvis to the bridge position.

3. Return to starting position with pelvis slightly lifted off the ground.

Perform the movement dynamically 15 times, then pause for 15 seconds before doing the next exercise.

Exercise 7

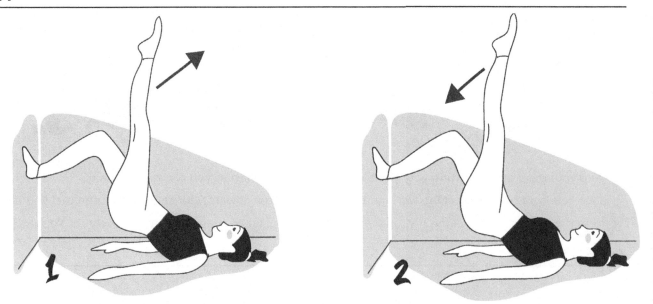

1. Hold the bridge position with one foot on the wall and the other raised overhead. Inhale and bring the leg slowly toward your forehead.

2. Exhale and bring the leg slowly toward the wall.

Perform the movement following the breath 15 times, then pause for 15 seconds and repeat the exercise with the other leg. Repeat 3 times.

Exercise 8

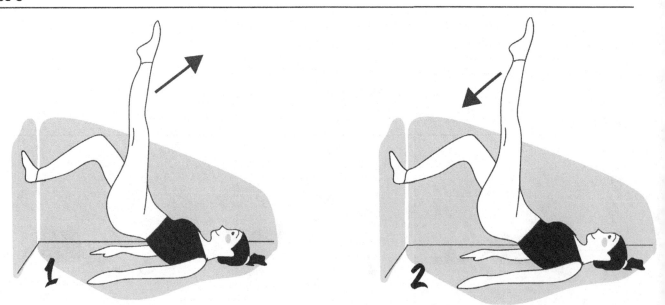

1. Hold the bridge position with one foot against the wall and the other raised overhead. Bring the leg toward your forehead.

2. Then bring the leg toward the wall.

Perform the movement dynamically 15 times, then pause for 15 seconds and repeat the exercise with the other leg. Repeat 3 times.

Exercise 9

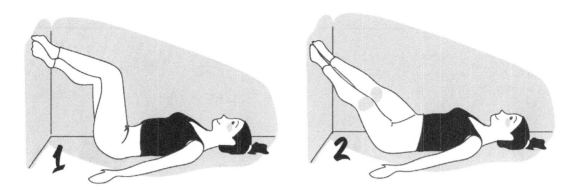

1. Rest your feet on the wall and keep your arms along your sides. Rotate your knees to the right without lifting your pelvis off the ground. Perform 3 deep breaths.

2. Rotate your knees to the left without lifting your pelvis off the ground. Perform 3 deep breaths.

Final relaxation

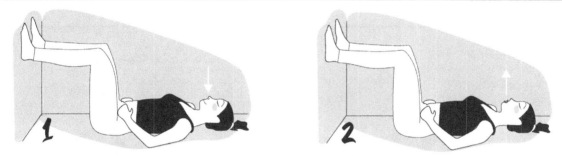

1. Rest your feet on the wall and keep your hands resting on your belly. Keep your eyes closed. Breathe in slowly through your nose until you feel your belly rise under your hands.

2. Exhale slowly with your mouth ajar and relax the muscles in your face. Repeat for 2 minutes.

Tip of the Day: Meal planning

An important aspect of getting back in shape is to never be caught unprepared at mealtime. When you are caught by hunger, you make impulsive decisions that lead you to unhealthy food choices. Preparing meals in advance is a strategy you can adopt to make sure you always have nutritious meals with the right energy intake.

The power is in your hands; you can be in control of your diet if you plan ahead.

WORKOUT DAY 3

Exercise 1

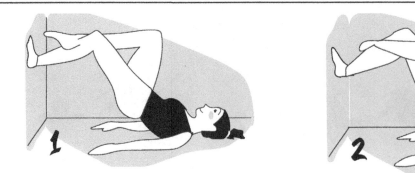

1. In the bridge position, keep one foot against the wall and the other crossed over your leg. Keep your arms along your sides. Take 3 long breaths.

2. Repeat with the other leg.

Perform the movement slowly 15 times.

Exercise 2

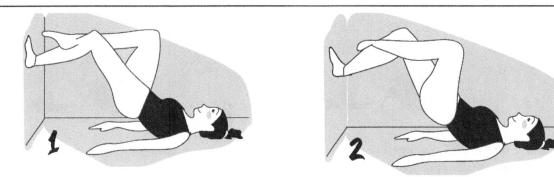

1. In the bridge position keep one foot against the wall and bring the other crossed over the leg.

2. Then switch feet.

Perform the movement 15 times dynamically (briskly, with energy), then pause for 15 seconds. Repeat 3 times.

Exercise 3

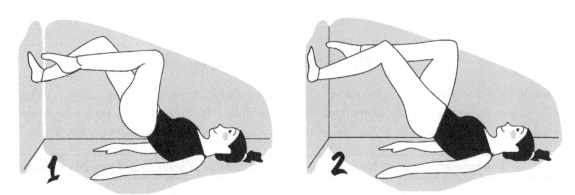

1. Hold the bridge position and contract the abdominals. Inhale and lift one foot. Exhale and press it against the wall.

2. Inhale and lift the other foot. Exhale and press it against the wall.

Perform the movement following the breath 15 times, then pause for 15 seconds. Repeat 3 times.

Exercise 4

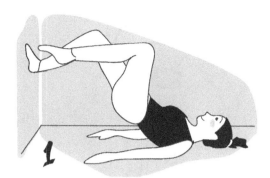 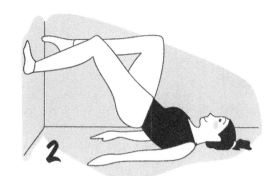

1. Hold the bridge position and contract your abs. Lift one foot and place it against the wall.

2. Lift the other foot and place it against the wall.

Perform the movement dynamically 15 times, then pause for 15 seconds. Repeat 3 times.

Exercise 5

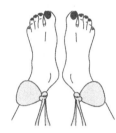

1. Use ankle weights. Keep your feet firm against the wall, your gaze upward, and your pelvis slightly off the ground.

2. Inhale and slowly lift the pelvis to a bridge position. Hold the position for a few seconds.

3. Exhale and return to the starting position with the pelvis slightly lifted off the ground.

4. Perform the movement slowly, following the breath, 15 times, then pause for 15. Repeat 3 times.

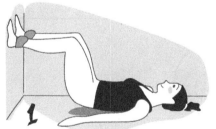 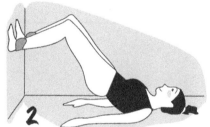 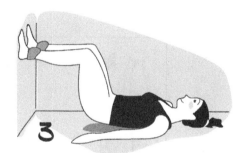

Exercise 6

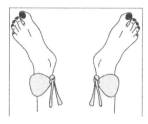

1. Use ankle weights. Keep your feet firm against the wall, toes pointed outward, your gaze upward, and your pelvis slightly off the ground.

2. Raise the pelvis to a bridge position.

3. Return to the starting position with the pelvis slightly lifted off the ground.

Perform the movement dynamically 15 times, then pause for 15. Repeat 3 times.

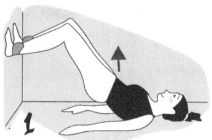 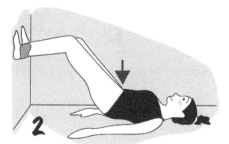 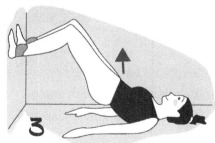

Exercise 7

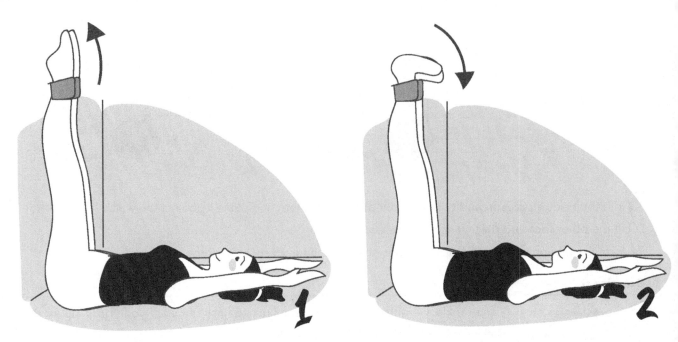

1. Keep your back on the floor and your outstretched legs resting against the wall. Keep your toes pointing upward. Take 3 slow breaths.

2. Then flex your feet to bring your toes downward and take 3 long breaths.

Perform the movement slowly 15 times, then pause for 15 seconds. Repeat 3 times.

Exercise 8

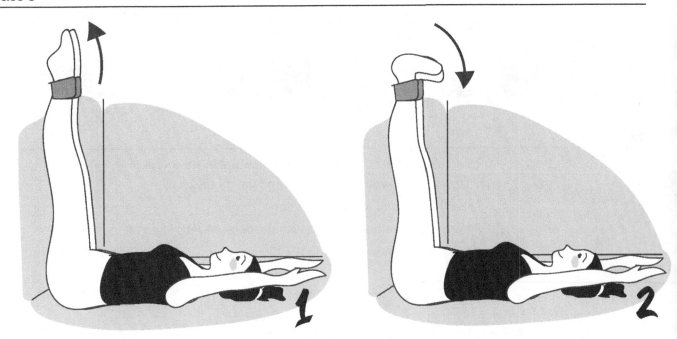

1. Keep your back on the floor and your outstretched legs resting against the wall. Point your toes upward.

2. Then flex your feet with energy.

Perform the movement dynamically 15 times, then pause for 15 seconds. Repeat 3 times.

Exercise 9

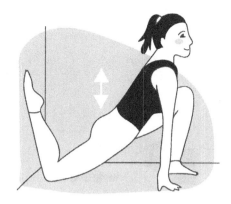

Perform a forward lunge and bend your right leg back and rest it against the wall. Keep your hands resting on the floor and look forward.

Raise and lower your pelvis 15 times. Then take a 15-second break. Repeat 3 times.

Final relaxation

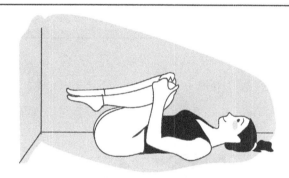

Lying on the floor, bring your knees to your chest and take long breaths for 3 minutes.

Tip of the Day: How to deflate the belly

A common problem for women at all stages of our lives is belly bloating. There are many causes: hormonal changes, hurried eating, stress, and the wrong choice of food. To have a flat belly, it is important to use fennel and anise herbal teas that naturally reduce stomach bloating. You can also try charcoal, which absorbs intestinal gas. Also, avoid skipping meals because arriving at the table hungry will lead you to eat too much too quickly. Finally, try to take long breaths and spend a few minutes meditating every day to regain serenity and banish stress.

Stress is the enemy of the waistline!

WORKOUT DAY 4

Exercise 1

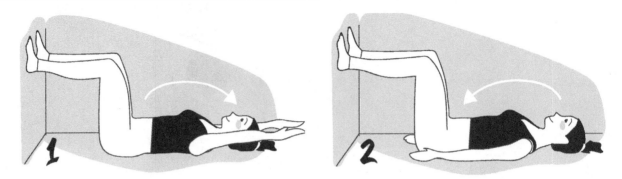

1. Keep your gaze upward and your feet firm against the wall. Exhale and bring your arms outstretched behind your head. Contract your abdominals.

2. Inhale and bring your arms slowly along your sides, following the breath.

Perform the movement following the breath 15 times, then pause for 15 seconds. Repeat 3 times.

Exercise 2

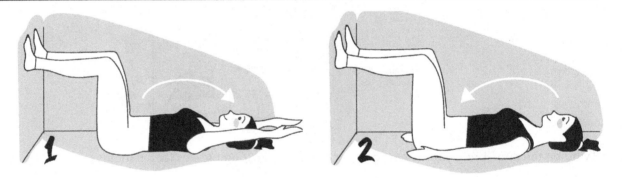

1. Keep your gaze upward and your feet firm against the wall. Bring your arms outstretched behind your head.

2. Then bring your arms along your sides.

Perform the movement dynamically (briskly, with energy) 15 times, then pause for 15 seconds. Repeat 3 times.

Exercise 3

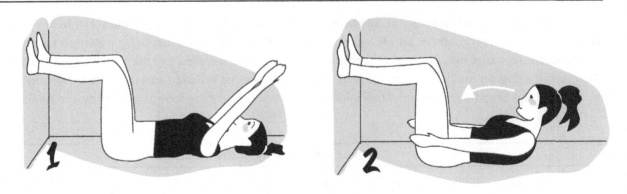

1. Keep your feet firm against the wall and your arms behind your head.

2. Bring your arms forward and lift your shoulders off the floor. Contract your abs and take 3 long breaths.

Perform the movement following the breath 15 times, then pause for 15 seconds. Repeat 3 times.

Exercise 4

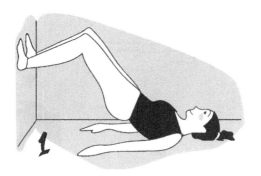 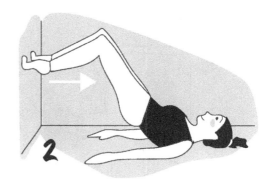

1. Hold the bridge position and contract your abs.

2. Lift your heels and press your toes against the wall.

Perform the movement dynamically 15 times, then pause for 15 seconds. Repeat 3 times.

Exercise 5

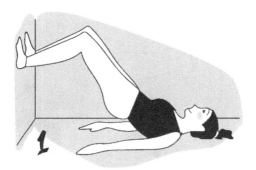 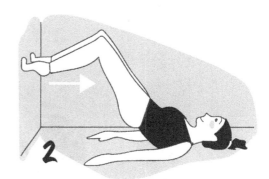

1. Hold the bridge position and contract your abs.

2. Lift your heels and press your toes against the wall. Hold this position while taking three long breaths.

Repeat the exercise slowly 3 times.

Exercise 6

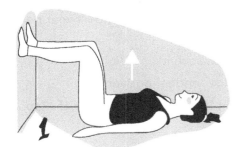 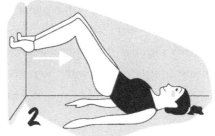 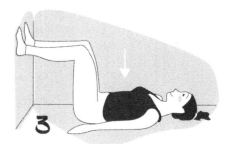

1. Keep your back on the floor, feet resting against the wall and look upward.

2. Lift your pelvis, lift your heels and press your toes against the wall.

3. Return to the starting position with your pelvis on the floor.

Perform the movement dynamically 15 times, then pause for 15 seconds. Repeat 3 times.

Exercise 7

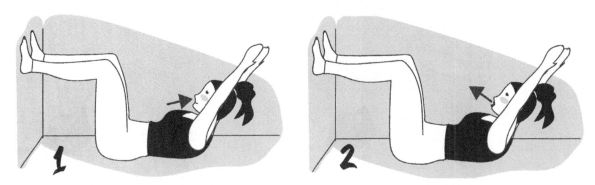

1. Keep your feet firmly against the wall, your arms close to your ears, your shoulders raised off the ground, and inhale deeply and slowly through your nose.

2. Slowly exhale through your mouth, holding the position.

Perform the movement following the breath 15 times, then pause for 15 seconds. Repeat 3 times.

Exercise 8

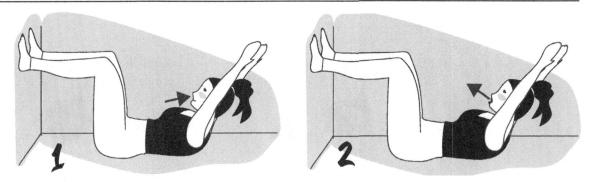

1. Keep your feet firmly against the wall, your arms close to your ears, your shoulders raised off the ground, and quickly inhale through your nose.

2. Slowly exhale through your mouth, holding the position.

Perform the movement dynamically 15 times, then pause for 15 seconds. Repeat 3 times.

Exercise 9

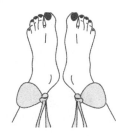

1. Use ankle weights. Keep feet firm against the wall, gaze upward, and lift your pelvis off the ground in the "bridge" position.

2. Lower the pelvis slightly. Hold the position for a few seconds.

3. Return to the starting position with the pelvis in the "bridge" position.

Perform the movement slowly, following the breath, 15 times, then pause for 15. Repeat 3 times.

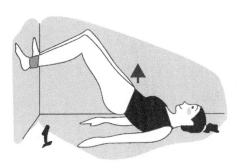
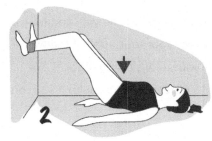
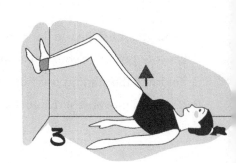

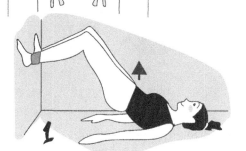

1. Use ankle weights. Keep feet firm against the wall, gaze upward, and lift your pelvis off the ground in the "bridge" position.

2. Lower the pelvis slightly.

3. Immediately return to the starting position with the pelvis in the "bridge" position.

Perform the movement dynamically 15 times, then pause for 15. Repeat 3 times.

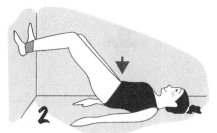
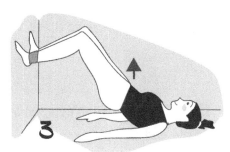

Final relaxation

Sitting on the floor with your legs crossed, reach one arm up from your waist and the other arm from your shoulder down your back, and try joining your hands. Hold the position for 1 minute and then switch arms.

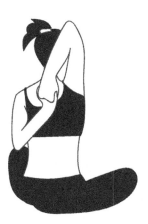

Tip of the Day: The cake that doesn't make you fat!

Do you think there is a dessert that is not fattening? The answer is yes! There are many recipes for cakes and cookies that are eggless, sugarless, flourless, suitable to satisfy the palate and very low in calories. But one particular cake manages to be fluffy and delicious and has very few calories: Water Cake. You can make it in 15 minutes (baking time 50 minutes) with water, sugar, oil, flour and yeast. Find several versions online. Don't stop trying and adapt your lifestyle and food choices to your goal of getting back in shape.

There are many alternatives for staying well without making sacrifices!

WORKOUT DAY 5

Exercise 1

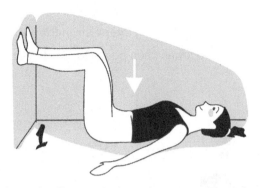 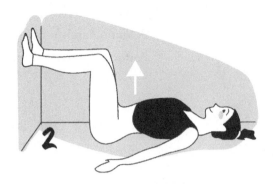

1. Keep your back on the floor, exhale and contract your abs.

2. Inhale and slowly lift your chest upward. Push your feet against the wall. Hold this position while taking three long breaths.

Repeat the exercise slowly 3 times.

Exercise 2

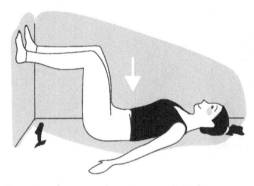 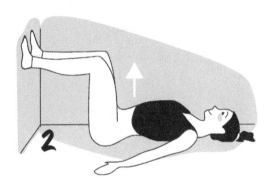

1. Keep your back on the floor and contract your abs.

2. Inhale and lift your chest upward. Push your feet up against the wall.

Return to position 1 and dynamically repeat the exercise 15 times, then take a 15-second break.

Repeat 3 times.

Exercise 3

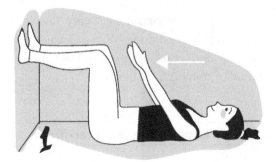 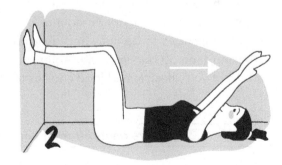

1. Keep your gaze upward and your feet firm against the wall. Exhale and bring your outstretched arms toward your knees without arching your back and contract your abdominals.

2. Inhale and bring your outstretched arms back over your head.

Perform the movement dynamically 15 times, then pause for 15 seconds. Repeat 3 times.

Exercise 4

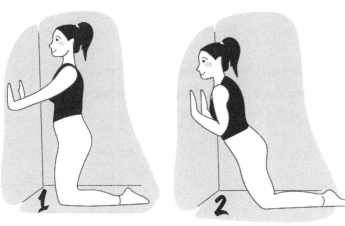

1. Kneel about 18" away from the wall (place a pillow under your knees if necessary) and gaze straight ahead. Inhale and place your hands against the wall.

2. Exhale and bend your arms.

Perform the movement slowly 15 times, then pause for 15 seconds. Repeat 3 times.

Exercise 5

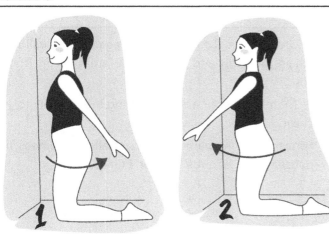

1.Kneel about 18" away from the wall (place a pillow under your knees if necessary) with your glutes contracted and look straight ahead. Inhale and swing your arms behind you.

2.Exhale and swing your arms forward to loosen your shoulders and neck.

Perform the movement dynamically 15 times, then pause for 15 seconds. Repeat 3 times.

Exercise 6

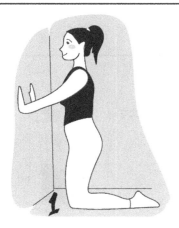 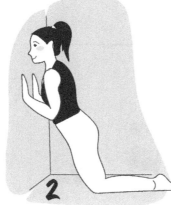

1.Kneel about a foot away from the wall (place a pillow under your knees if necessary) and gaze forward. Inhale and place your hands against the wall.

2.Exhale and bend your arms.

Perform the movement dynamically 15 times, then pause for 15 seconds. Repeat 3 times.

Exercise 7

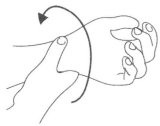

Pause and loosen both wrists before continuing.

Circle your wrists both to the right and left.

Perform a gentle massage.

Exercise 8

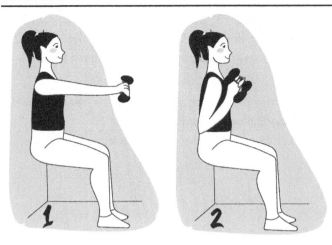

1. Use weights. Lean your back against the wall in the "chair" position, inhale and extend your arms in front of you.

2. Exhale and bring the weights to your chest.

Perform the movement slowly 15 times, then pause for 15 seconds. Repeat 3 times.

Exercise 9

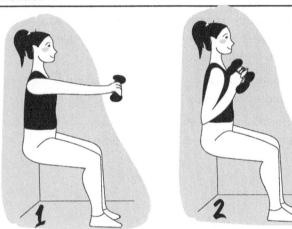

1. Use weights. Lean your back against the wall in the "chair" position and stretch your arms out in front of you.

2. Then bend your arms and bring the weights to your chest.

Perform the movement dynamically 15 times, then pause for 15 seconds. Repeat 3 times.

Exercise 10

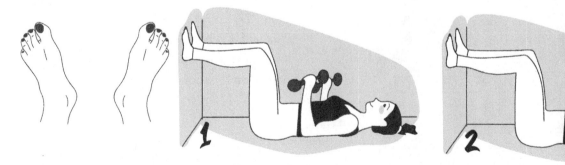

1. Rest your feet against the wall, spaced apart, with your toes pointed outward. Keep your gaze facing up. Use weights and bend your arms close to your chest.

2. Then extend your arms overhead.

Perform the movement quickly 15 times, then pause for 15 seconds. Repeat 3 times.

Exercise 11

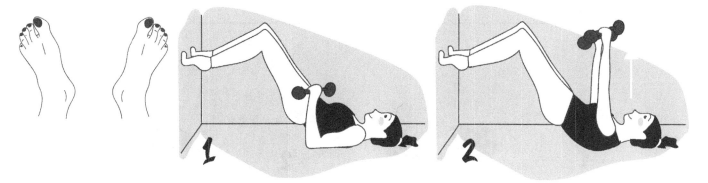

1. Rest your feet against the wall, spaced apart, with toes facing outward. Raise your hips into the bridge position and lift your heels off the wall. Keep your gaze upward. Use weights and bend your arms close to your chest.

2. Then extend your arms overhead.

Perform the movement quickly 15 times, then pause for 15 seconds. Repeat 3 times.

Final relaxation

Sitting on the floor with legs crossed, extend one arm across your body, grasp the elbow, and gently pull the arm toward the torso. Hold the position for 30 seconds and then repeat, changing sides.

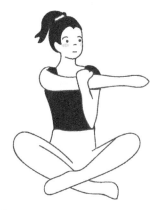

Tip of the Day: Why is it necessary to drink so much water?

It is well known that drinking plenty of water is good for you and is strongly suggested, especially when dieting or if you practice sports, but do you really know the benefits of water? Knowing why it is important is a strong incentive to really drink up to eight 8-oz glasses of water a day; two of the reasons are hydration and appetite control. Water can help keep the body hydrated, but it can also reduce the feeling of hunger. Sometimes thirst can be confused with hunger. Drinking plenty of water can help reduce the appetite and avoid overeating or making unhealthy food choices. Drinking water will increase the metabolism, thus facilitating the weight loss process; water serves to eliminate waste and toxins from the body through urine and sweat. Finally, drinking a lot can trick the body as it produces a sense of satiety.

Drinking helps with weight loss and maintaining a clean and healthy body.

WORKOUT DAY 6

Exercise 1

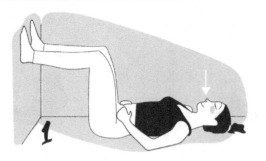 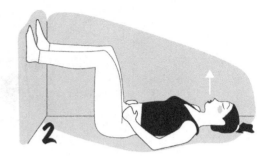

1. Rest your feet on the wall and rest your hands on your belly. Keep your eyes closed. Breathe in slowly through your nose until you feel your belly rise under your hands.

2. Exhale slowly with your mouth ajar and relax the muscles in your face. Repeat for 2 minutes.

Exercise 2

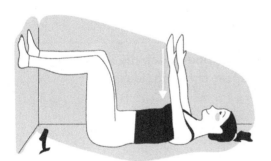 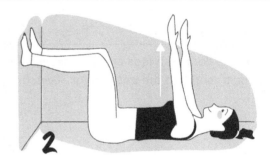

1. Keep your gaze upward and your feet firm against the wall. Raise your outstretched arms toward the ceiling with shoulders firmly on the floor and palms facing inward.

2. Stretch your arms upward by pulling your shoulders off the ground, without arching your back, then return with your shoulders resting on the ground.

Perform the movement slowly following the breath 15 times, then pause for 15 seconds. Repeat 3 times.

Exercise 3

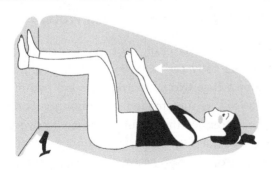 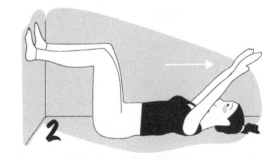

1. Keep your gaze upward and your feet firm against the wall. Bring your outstretched arms toward your knees without arching your back.

2. Keeping your arms straight, bring them over your head, past your gaze.

Perform the movement dynamically 15 times, then pause for 15 seconds. Repeat 3 times.

Exercise 4

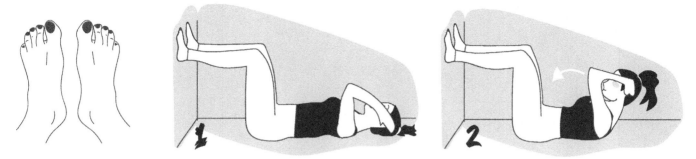

1. Place your feet close together, firm against the wall, and your hands behind your head.
2. Raise your shoulders and contract your abdominal muscles. Perform the movement quickly 20 times, then pause for 5 seconds. Repeat 3 times.

Exercise 5

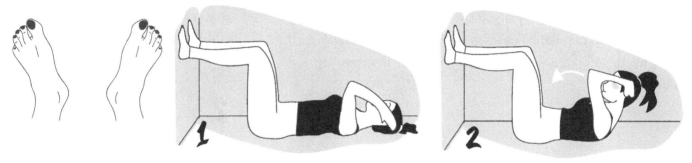

1. Place your feet hip-width apart, firm against the wall, with your hands behind your head.
2. Raise your shoulders and contract your abdominal muscles. Perform the movement quickly 20 times, then pause for 5 seconds. Repeat 3 times.

Exercise 6

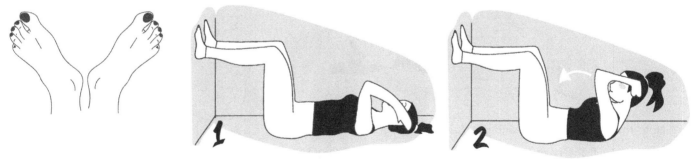

1. Rest your feet against the wall, joined together, with your toes open, and hold your hands behind the back of your head.

2. Raise your shoulders and keep your abdominal muscles contracted.

Perform the movement quickly 15 times, then pause for 15'' seconds. Repeat 3 times.

Exercise 7

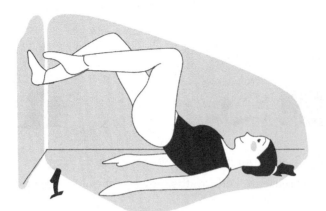

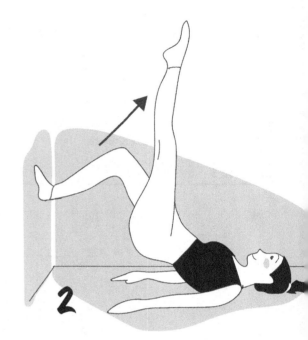

1. Hold the bridge position with one foot resting on the wall.
2. Inhale and contract your glutes and abs; hold the position for 3 slow breaths. Exhale and straighten the leg toward the ceiling, then return to the starting position without touching the wall.

Pause for 15 seconds and repeat the exercise with the other leg.

Repeat 3 times.

Exercise 8

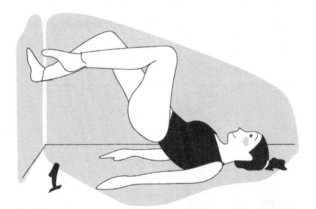

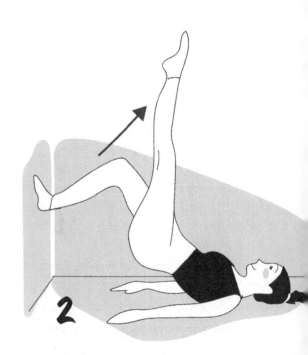

1. Hold the bridge position with one foot resting on the wall.
2. Inhale and tighten your abs and glutes. Exhale and straighten the leg upward; return to the starting position without resting the foot on the wall.

Perform the movement dynamically 15 times, then pause for 15 seconds.

Repeat the exercise with the other leg.

Repeat 3 times.

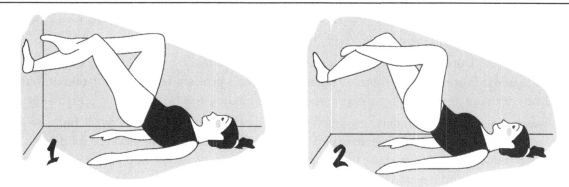

1. In the bridge position keep one foot against the wall and cross the other over the supporting leg. Allow your knee to fall open so your hip is as wide as possible.

2. Then switch feet, crossing the other foot over the leg and opening the other hip.

Perform the movement 15 times in a dynamic but gentle manner.

Final relaxation

Standing with your legs against the wall and rest your hands on a ball on the floor. Hold the position for 1 minute while taking long breaths.

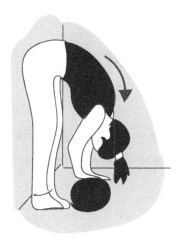

Tip of the Day: How to reduce hunger pangs

"It's best to chew each bite at least 33 times," an old aunt of mine had recommended. And she was right!

Chewing a lot starts the digestion process on food already in the mouth, thanks to the digestive power of saliva. A well-chewed meal reduces abdominal bloating problems. Chewing slowly also allows you to savor food and identify flavors. In addition, chewing a lot sends satiety impulses to the brain that help keep the amount of food consumed under control.

Chew each bite 33 times and see how different each meal tastes.

PAUSE DAY 7: Why is taking a break important?

This is a day dedicated to resting. Taking a break is essential during a training program to get fit and lose weight. I have included 4 rest days in this program for the following benefits:

• Muscle regeneration: During exercises, muscles suffer micro-injuries. By taking a break, the body has time to repair these injuries. This allows the muscles to strengthen and prepare for the next workout. Muscle overload puts your body at risk of injury. Resting allows tissues to stay healthy and be in better shape the next day.

• Mental regeneration: Rest is not only important for the body but also for the mind because during sleep, relaxation and meditation, the brain processes information gathered over time and consolidates it into memory. Relaxation also reduces levels of cortisol, the stress hormone, and allows for decreased anxiety and promotes a good mood. A healthy mind is a creative, focused and vibrant mind.

So enjoy your day off!!!

WORKOUT DAY 8

Exercise 1

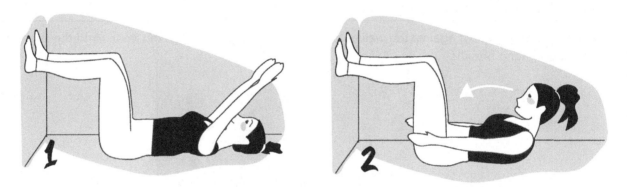

1. Keep your feet firm against the wall and your arms on the floor over your head.

2. Bring your arms outstretched forward and lift your shoulders off the floor. Contract your abs and take 3 long breaths.

Perform the movement following the breath 15 times, then pause for 15 seconds. Repeat 3 times.

Exercise 2

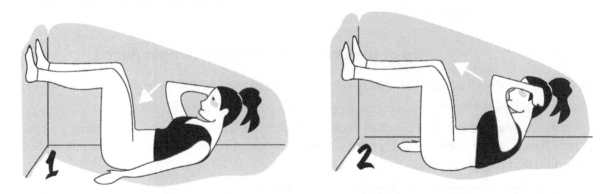

1. Keep your feet firmly against the wall with one arm behind your head. Bring your elbow toward the opposite knee and take a long breath.

2. Then bring your other arm behind your head. Bring your elbow toward the opposite knee and take a long breath.

Perform the movement following the breath 15 times, then pause for 15 seconds. Repeat 3 times.

Exercise 3

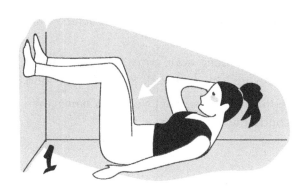 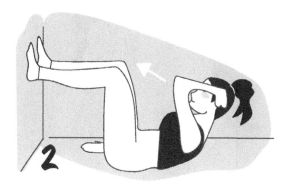

1. Keep your feet firmly against the wall and one arm behind your head. Bring your elbow toward the opposite knee.

2. Then bring your other arm behind your head. Bring your elbow toward the opposite knee.

Perform the movement dynamically (briskly, with energy) 15 times, then pause for 15 seconds. Repeat 3 times.

Exercise 4

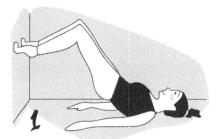 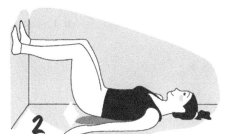 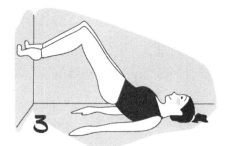

1. Inhale and hold the bridge position with heels raised; contract your abs and take 3 long breaths.

2. Exhale and lower your pelvis without touching the floor. Hold this position while taking 3 long breaths.

3. Inhale and return to the starting position, contract the abdominals, and take 3 long breaths.

Repeat the exercise slowly 3 times.

Exercise 5

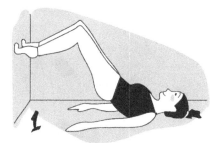 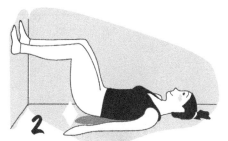 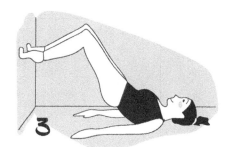

1. Inhale and go into the bridge position with heels raised.

2. Exhale and lower the pelvis without touching the ground.

3. Inhale and return to the starting position.

Perform the movement dynamically 15 times, then pause for 15 seconds. Repeat 3 times.

Exercise 6

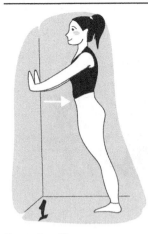 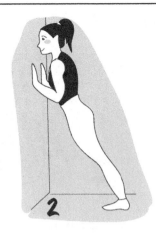

1. Inhale and place your hands against the wall, leaning forward, with your glutes contracted. Take three long breaths.

2. Exhale to bend your arms until your face is close to the wall. Do not arch your back. Perform three long breaths.

3. Perform the movement slowly 15 times, then pause for 15 seconds. Repeat 3 times.

Exercise 7

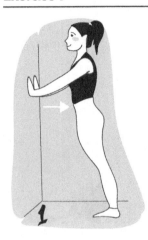 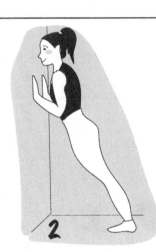

1. Place your hands against the wall, leaning forward, with your glutes contracted.

2. Bend your arms until your face is close to the wall. Do not arch your back.

Perform the movement dynamically 15 times, then pause for 15 seconds. Repeat 3 times.

Exercise 8

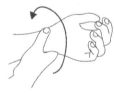

Pause and loosen both wrists before continuing.

Roll your wrists to the right and left.

Perform a gentle massage.

Exercise 9

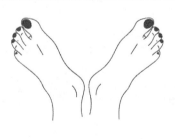 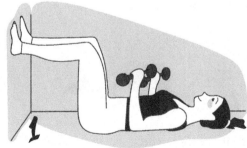 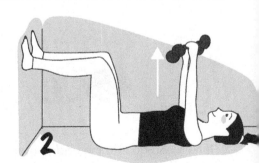

1. Rest your feet against the wall, toes pointed outward. Keep your gaze upward. Bend your arms at your sides with weights above your chest.

2. Then extend your arms overhead.

Perform the movement quickly 15 times, then pause for 15 seconds. Repeat 3 times.

Exercise 10

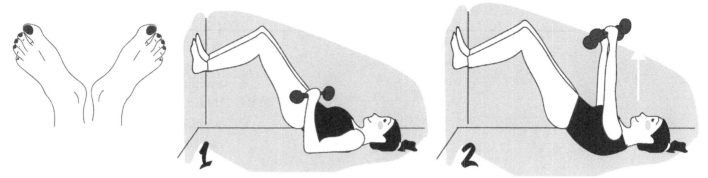

1. Rest your feet against the wall, toes pointed outward. Lift your pelvis and gaze upward.

2. Bend your arms at your sides with weights above your chest.

3. Then extend your arms overhead.

4. Perform the movement quickly 15 times, then pause for 15 seconds. Repeat 3 times.

Final relaxation

Lying on the floor with your legs pulled into your chest, place your hands on your knees and move your legs side to side, massaging your back into the floor. Then make circular movements. Repeat slowly for 1 minute.

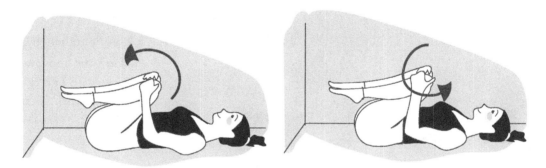

Tip of the Day: Which snacks to choose

Stress, fatigue, and even boredom can lead to the desire to eat something when it's not mealtime. Often, however, what is easy to eat even while standing and without the need for preparation is unhealthy and fattening food, such as chocolate, cookies, or a slice of bread. Prevent these mistakes by keeping healthy and nutritious food on hand such as apple slices, pre-washed grapes, almonds, sliced carrots, and grape tomatoes.

A well-chosen snack is a source of vitamins, fiber and potassium.

WORKOUT DAY 9

Exercise 1

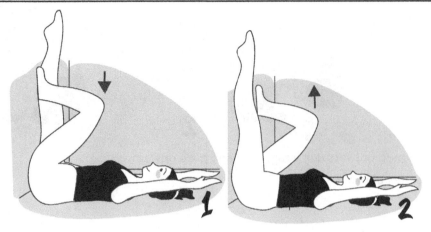

1. Rest your outstretched legs against the wall with your back flat on the floor. Flex one leg slowly, then extend it.

2. Flex the other leg slowly then extend it.

Perform the movement slowly 15 times, then pause for 15 seconds. Repeat 3 times.

Exercise 2

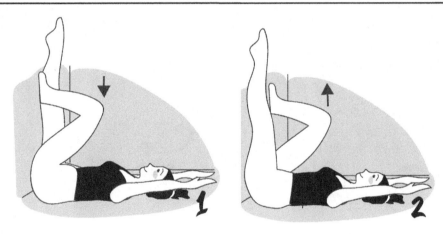

1. Rest your outstretched legs against the wall with your back flat on the floor. Flex one leg, then extend it.

2. Flex the other leg, then extend it.

Perform the movement dynamically (briskly, with energy) 15 times, then pause for 15 seconds. Repeat 3 times.

Exercise 3

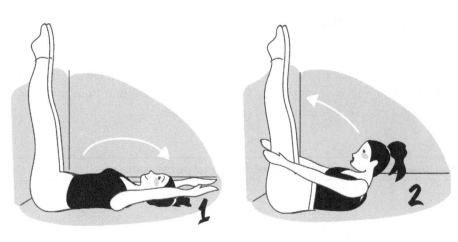

1. Rest your outstretched legs against the wall with your back flat on the floor. Inhale and raise your arms over your head.

2. Exhale and bring your arms to your thighs while lifting your shoulders off the floor.

Perform the movement slowly 15 times, then pause for 15 seconds. Repeat 3 times.

Exercise 4

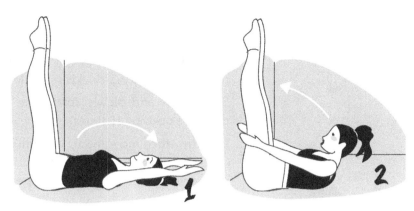

1. Rest your outstretched legs against the wall with your back flat on the floor. Inhale and raise your arms above your head.

2. Exhale and bring your arms to your thighs, lifting your shoulders off the floor.

Perform the movement dynamically 15 times, then pause for 15 seconds. Repeat 3 times.

Exercise 5

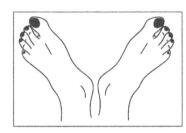

1. Keep your feet against the wall with your toes facing outward. Inhale and go into the bridge position with heels raised.

2. Exhale and lower your pelvis without touching the floor while also lowering your heels.

3. Inhale and return to the starting position.

Perform the movement slowly 15 times, then pause for 15 seconds. Repeat 3 times.

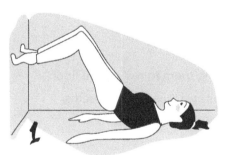 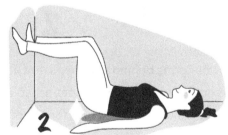 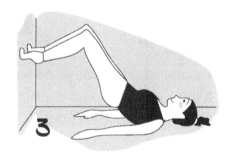

Exercise 6

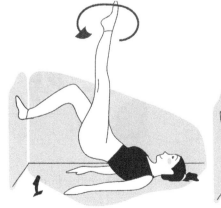 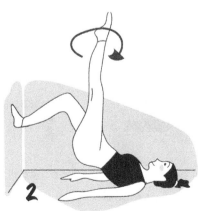

1. Place one foot against the wall and lift your pelvis off the ground. With the other leg, make 15 clockwise circles in the air.

2. Reverse directions and make 15 counterclockwise circles in the air.

Perform the movement slowly with both legs, then pause for 15 seconds. Repeat 3 times.

Exercise 7

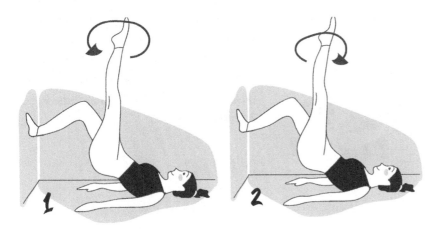

1. Place one foot against the wall and lift your pelvis off the ground. Slowly rotate the outstretched leg clockwise 15 times.

2. Reverse and slowly rotate the leg counterclockwise 15 times.

Perform the movement dynamically (briskly, with energy) with both legs, then pause for 15 seconds. Repeat 3 times.

Exercise 8

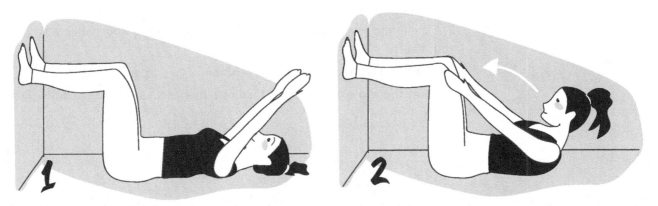

1. Firmly plant your feet on the wall with your arms behind your head, not allowing them to rest on the floor.

2. Bring your arms forward and lift your shoulders off the floor. Contract your abs and take 3 long breaths.

Perform the movement following the breath 15 times, then pause for 15 seconds. Repeat 3 times.

Exercise 9

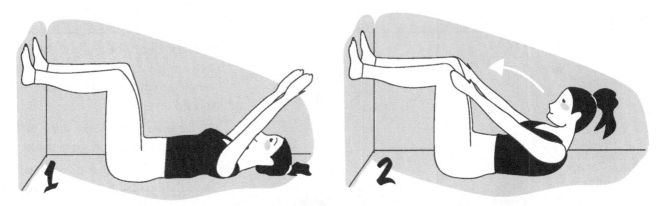

1. Firmly plant your feet on the wall with your arms behind your head, not allowing them to rest on the floor.

2. Bring your arms outstretched forward and lift your shoulders off the floor.

Perform the movement dynamically 15 times, then pause for 15 seconds. Repeat 3 times.

Exercise 10

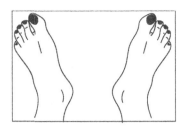

1. Place your feet hip-width apart against the wall.

2. Inhale and bring your arms over your head.

3. Exhale, lifting your shoulders slightly and bending your arms towards your chest.

4. Inhale and touch your knees with your hands. Contract your abs and take 3 long breaths.

Perform the movement following the breath 15 times, then pause for 15 seconds. Repeat 3 times.

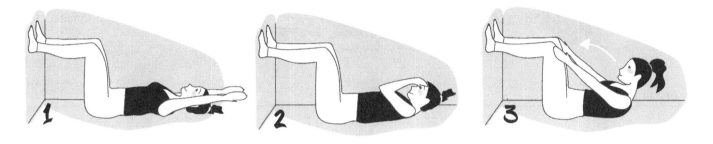

Final relaxation

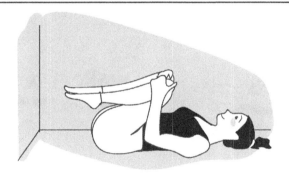

Lying on the floor, bend your knees to your chest and take long breaths for 3 minutes.

Tip of the Day: Involuntary exercise

Escalators, elevators, and moving walkways have sped up our lives but have also greatly reduced our involuntary exercise. Choosing to take the elevator instead of walking decreases the day's aerobic activity. Aerobic activity works your heart and lungs and is a great stress reliever. I recommend that you take every opportunity to walk and thus take advantage of involuntary exercise, which is available to everyone every day!

Next time, don't take the elevator: Walk!

WORKOUT DAY 10

Exercise 1

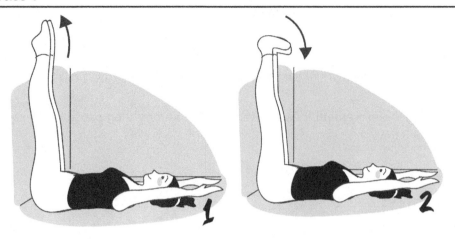

1. Rest your outstretched legs against the wall, your back flat on the floor. Flex one foot slowly, then point it.

2. Flex the other foot slowly, then point it.

Perform the movement slowly 15 times, then pause for 15 seconds. Repeat 3 times.

Exercise 2

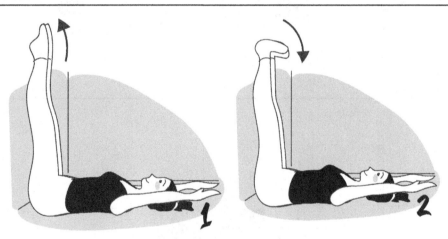

1. Rest your outstretched legs against the wall, your back flat on the floor. Flex one foot, then point it.

2. Flex the other foot, then point it. Perform the movement dynamically 15 times, then pause for 15 seconds. Repeat 3 times.

Exercise 3

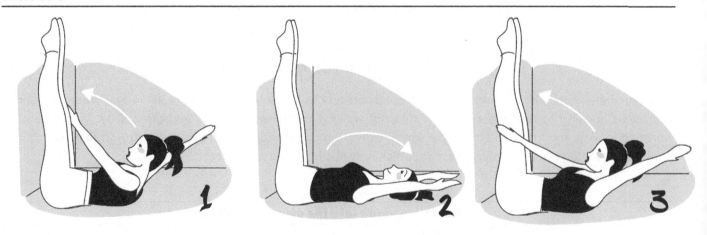

1. Rest your outstretched legs against the wall, your back flat on the floor. Exhale, lifting your shoulders off the floor, and touch your left hand to your right knee.

2. Inhale and return your back to the floor.

3. Exhale and repeat on the other side.

Perform the movement slowly 15 times, then pause for 15 seconds. Repeat 3 times.

Exercise 4

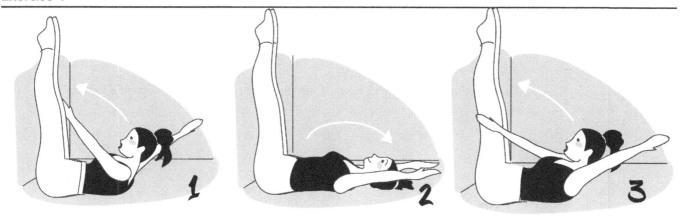

1. Rest your outstretched legs
   against the wall, your back flat on the floor. Exhale, lifting your shoulders off the floor, and touch your left hand to your right knee.
2. Inhale and return your back to the floor.
3. Exhale and repeat on the other side.

Perform the movement dynamically 15 times, then pause for 15 seconds. Repeat 3 times.

Exercise 5

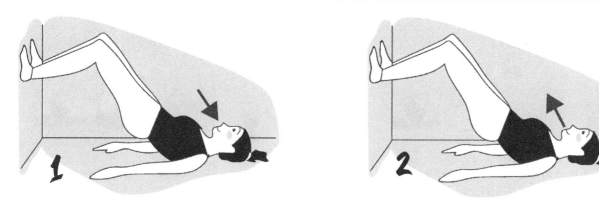

1. Keep your feet firm against the wall in the bridge position with your arms along your sides. Inhale deeply through the nose.
2. Hold the position and exhale deeply through your mouth.

Perform the movement following the breath 15 times, then pause for 15 seconds. Repeat 3 times.

Exercise 6

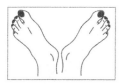

1. Use weights. Keep your feet firm against the wall, heels together and toes apart, and bend your arms toward your torso.
2. Extend the arms.

Perform the movement 15 times, then pause for 15 seconds. Repeat 3 times.

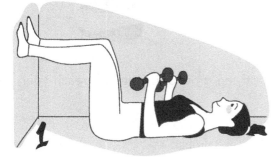

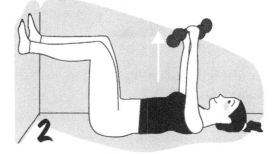

Exercise 7

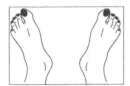

1. Use weights. Keep your feet firm against the wall, hip-width apart with toes facing out, and bend your arms toward your torso.

2. Extend the arms.

Perform the movement 15 times, then pause for 15 seconds. Repeat 3 times.

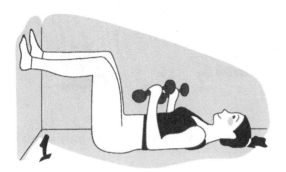 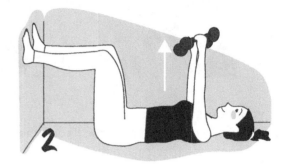

Exercise 8

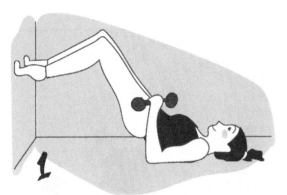 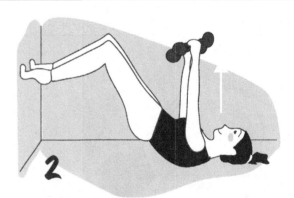

1. Keeping your feet firm against the wall with your heels lifted, go into the bridge position. Use weights and keep your arms flexed close to your sides.

2. Extend your arms without coming down from the bridge position.

Perform the movement dynamically (briskly, with energy) 15 times, then pause for 15 seconds. Repeat 3 times.

Exercise 9

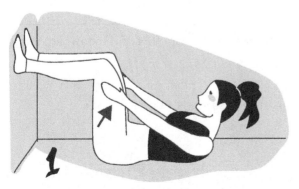 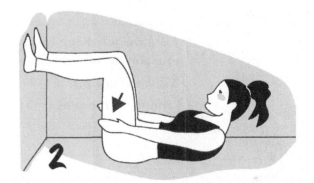

1. Keep your feet firm against the wall and your shoulders raised off the ground. Exhale and reach your arms towards your knees.

2. Hold the position. Inhale and bring your arms toward the floor.

Perform the movement slowly 15 times, then pause for 15 seconds. Repeat 3 times.

Exercise 10

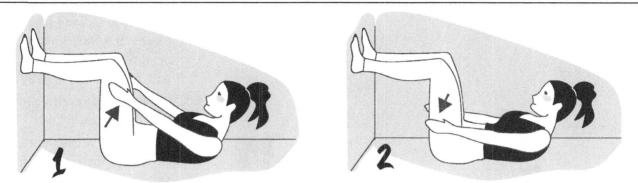

1. Keep your feet firm against the wall and your shoulders raised off the ground. Reach your arms towards your knees.

2. Quickly lower your arms toward the floor without touching it.

Perform the arm movement quickly 15 times, then pause for 15 seconds. Repeat 3 times.

Final relaxation

Standing with your legs against the wall, resting your hands on the ball on the floor. Hold the position for 1 minute while taking long breaths.

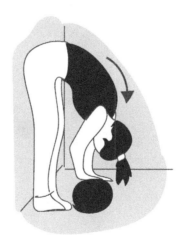

Tip of the Day: Anti-cellulite posture

Cellulite is a problem that afflicts all women. Sometimes the cause is the wrong diet (fat, salt, and sugar), but often the reason lies in poor posture. Do you work long hours at the computer? Are you on the couch a lot? Do you read books? To avoid accumulating cellulite on your legs and hips, be careful never to keep your legs crossed when sitting and avoid tight pants and high heels. These simple steps are important for the well-being of your tissues.

Avoid keeping your legs crossed!

WORKOUT DAY 11

Exercise 1

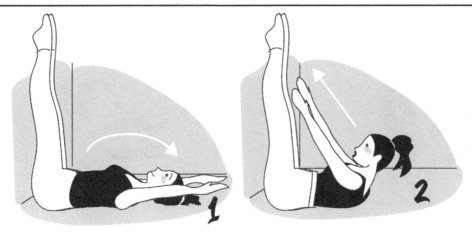

1. Rest your outstretched legs against the wall, your back flat on the floor. Inhale and raise your arms over your head.

2. Exhale and reach your arms toward your toes.

Perform the movement slowly 15 times, then pause for 15 seconds. Repeat 3 times.

Exercise 2

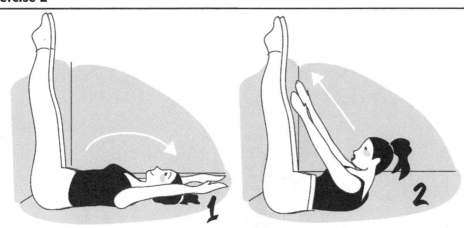

1. Rest your outstretched legs against the wall, your back flat on the floor. Raise your arms over your head.

2. Reach your arms toward your toes.

Perform the movement dynamically 15 times, then pause for 15 seconds. Repeat 3 times.

Exercise 3

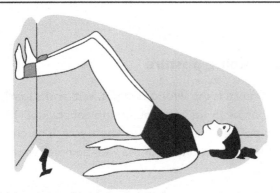 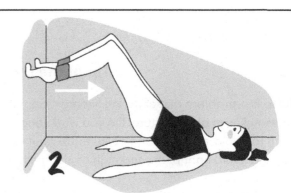

1. Use ankle weights. Hold the bridge position and contract your abs.

2. Lift your heels and press your toes against the wall. Hold this position while taking three long breaths.

Repeat the exercise slowly 3 times.

Exercise 4

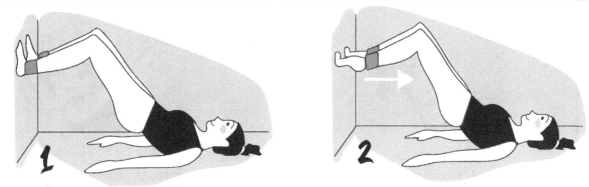

1. Use ankle weights. Hold the bridge position and contract your abs.

2. Lift your heels and press your toes against the wall.

Perform the movement dynamically 15 times, then pause for 15 seconds. Repeat 3 times.

Exercise 5

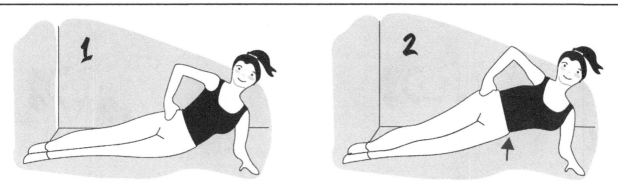

1. Lie on your side, propped up on one forearm. Keep your other arm resting on your side.

2. Lift your hip off the floor and hold the position for three long breaths.

Perform the movement slowly 15 times, then pause for 15 seconds. Repeat on the opposite side.

Exercise 6

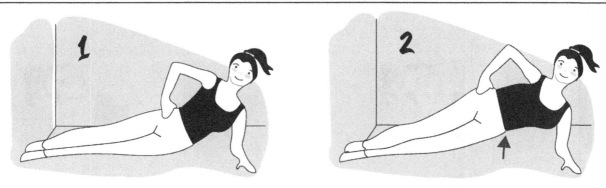

1. Lie on your side with your weight on your arm on the ground. Keep your other arm resting on your side.

2. Lift your hip off the floor and then return to the ground position.

Perform the movement dynamically (briskly, with energy) 15 times, then pause for 15 seconds. Repeat on the opposite side.

Exercise 7

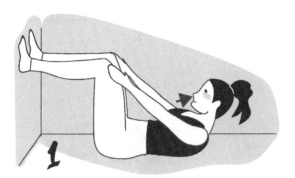 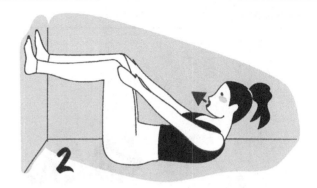

1. Keep your feet firm against the wall, your hands at your knees. Inhale deeply through your nose.

2. Hold the position and exhale deeply through your mouth.

Perform the movement following the breath 15 times, then pause for 15 seconds. Repeat 3 times.

Exercise 8

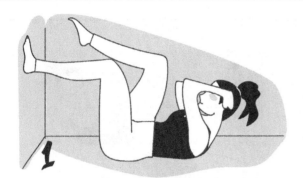 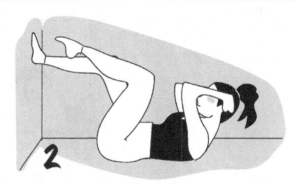

1. Keep your feet firmly against the wall, your hands behind your head. Inhale and lift your right knee.

2. Exhale and lift your left knee.

Perform the movement following the breath 15 times, then pause for 15 seconds. Repeat 3 times.

Exercise 9

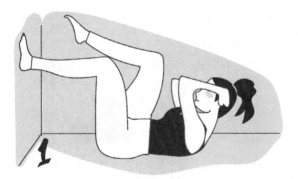 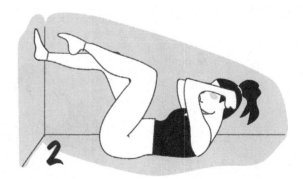

1. Keep your feet firm against the wall, your hands behind your head. Lift your right knee and touch it with the opposite elbow.

2. Lift your left knee and touch it with the opposite elbow.

Perform the movement dynamically 15 times, then pause for 15 seconds. Repeat 3 times.

Exercise 10

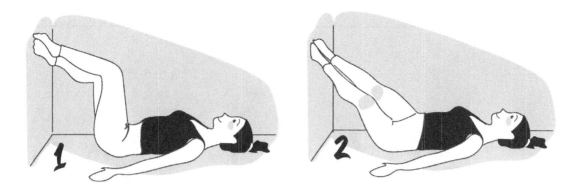

1. Rest your feet on the wall and keep your arms along your sides. Rotate your knees to the right without lifting your pelvis off the ground. Perform 3 deep breaths.

2. Rotate your knees to the left without lifting your pelvis off the ground. Perform 3 deep breaths.

Final relaxation

Sitting on the floor with your legs crossed, reach one arm over your shoulder and the other up from your lower back, and try to join your hands behind your back. Hold the position for 1 minute and then repeat by changing sides.

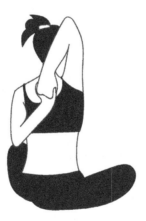

Tip of the Day: Procrastination is the enemy

One of the reasons for stress and frustration is the habit of not doing what one would like to do and always putting it off until tomorrow. This is a common evil for people and causes loss of self-esteem and non-achievement of goals.

In order not to fall into the temptation of always putting things off until tomorrow, one ploy is to immediately do the small tasks that come up day by day, such as paying bills, making a difficult phone call, or making a doctor's appointment. This will relieve your days and make you feel lighter and more confident – crucial components for following this Wall Pilates program to the end.

Don't put off until tomorrow what you can do today.

WORKOUT DAY 12

Exercise 1

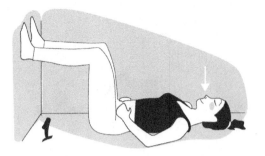 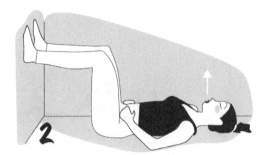

1. Place your feet on the wall and rest your hands on your belly. Keep your eyes closed. Breathe in slowly through your nose until you feel your belly rise under your hands.

2. Exhale slowly with your mouth ajar and relax the muscles in your face. Repeat for 2 minutes.

Exercise 2

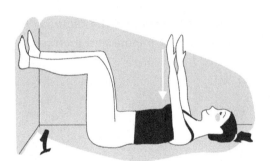 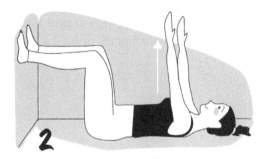

1. Keep your gaze upward and your feet firm against the wall. Maintain slow breathing and relaxed facial muscles. Bring arms outstretched towards the ceiling, with shoulders firmly on the floor and palms facing inward.

2. Stretch your arms upward by pulling your shoulders off the ground, without arching your back, then return with your shoulders resting on the ground.

Perform the movement dynamically 15 times, then pause for 15 seconds. Repeat 3 times.

Exercise 3

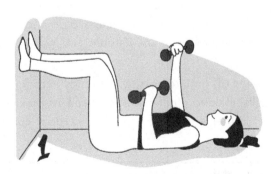 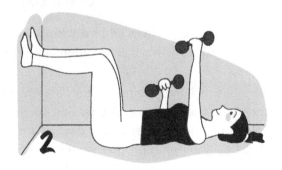

1. Use weights. Keep your feet firm against the wall, hip-width apart. Bend one arm toward the torso while extending the other arm overhead.

2. Switch arms.

Perform the movement dynamically 15 times, then pause for 15 seconds. Repeat 3 times.

Exercise 4

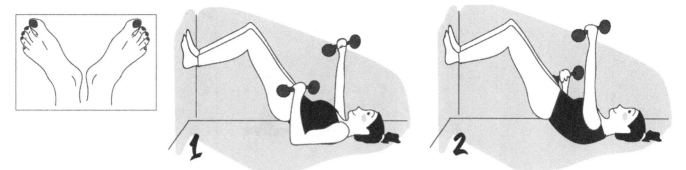

1. Use weights. Keep feet together and firm against the wall, heels touching and toes facing outward. Go into the bridge position. Bend one arm toward the torso while extending the other arm overhead.

2. Switch arms without coming down from the bridge position.

Perform the movement dynamically 15 times, then pause for 15 seconds. Repeat 3 times.

Exercise 5

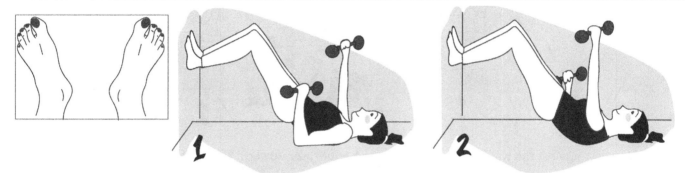

1. Use weights. Keep your feet slightly apart and firm against the wall. Go into the bridge position. Bend one arm toward the torso while extending the other arm overhead.

2. Switch arms without coming down from the bridge position.

Perform the movement dynamically 15 times, then pause for 15 seconds. Repeat 3 times.

Exercise 6

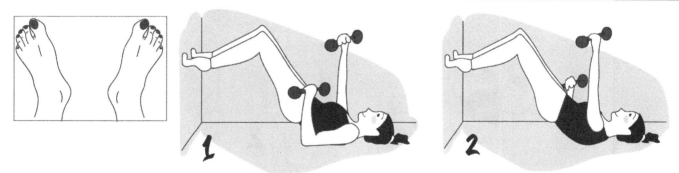

1. Use weights. Keep feet slightly apart and firm against the wall. Lift your heels. Go into the bridge position. Bend one arm toward the torso while extending the other arm overhead.

2. Switch arms without coming down from the bridge position.

Perform the movement dynamically 15 times, then pause for 15 seconds. Repeat 3 times.

Exercise 7

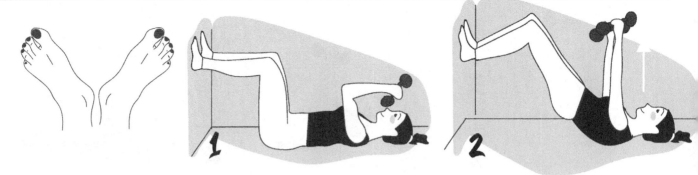

1. Rest your feet against the wall, toes facing out. Keep your gaze upward. Use weights. Inhale and bend your elbows so your hands are close to your forehead.

2. Then exhale, extend arms overhead and go into the bridge position.

Perform the movement slowly following the breath 15 times, then pause for 15 seconds. Repeat 3 times.

Exercise 8

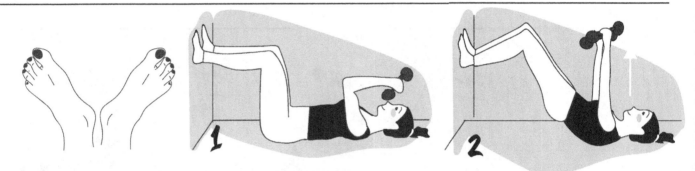

1. Rest your feet against the wall, toes facing out. Keep your gaze upward. Use weights. Bend your arms so your hands are close to your forehead.

2. Then extend your arms overhead and go into the bridge position.

Perform the movement dynamically (briskly, with energy) 15 times, then pause for 15 seconds. Repeat 3 times.

Exercise 9

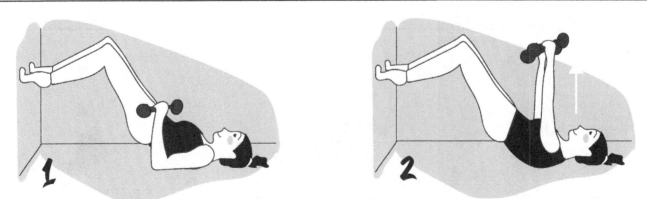

1. Keeping your feet firm against the wall with your heels lifted, go into the bridge position. Use weights and keep your arms bent close to your sides.

2. Extend your arms to the ceiling without coming down from the bridge position.

Perform the movement dynamically 15 times, then pause for 15 seconds. Repeat 3 times.

Exercise 10

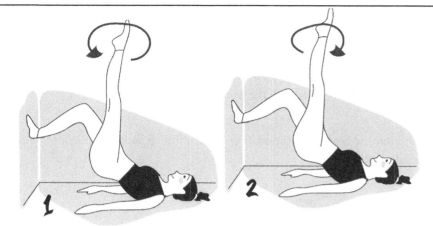

1.Lean one foot against the wall and lift your pelvis off the ground. Slowly rotate the other leg, pointed towards the ceiling, clockwise 15 times.

2.Slowly rotate the leg counterclockwise 15 times.

Perform the movement with both legs, then pause for 15 seconds. Repeat 3 times.

Final relaxation

Lying on the floor, bend your knees to your chest and take long breaths for 3 minutes.

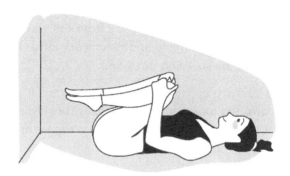

Tip of the Day: To-do list

Getting organized is the first thing you need to do to manage your time and prevent it from managing you.

Here is a sample list you can use to compile your personal list. Don't forget to include times for breaks and gratitude.

7 a.m.: wake up and meditate; 7:30 a.m. Breakfast; 8 a.m. Work; 10 a.m. Break and snack; 12 p.m. lunch with a friend; 2 p.m. Work; 4 p.m. Break with a snack and pleasure call; 6 p.m. Pilates at the wall; 6:30 p.m. Shower and read a book; 8 p.m. Light dinner and movie. 11 p.m. Bedtime.

Organization is a good way not to get overwhelmed!

WORKOUT DAY 13

Exercise 1

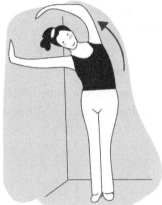

Stand at an arm's length away from the wall and place your right arm on it at shoulder height. Inhale and reach your left arm toward the wall, over your head. Perform three long breaths. Return to the standing position.

Perform the movement slowly 15 times, then pause for 15 seconds. Repeat 3 times, then repeat on the other side.

Exercise 2

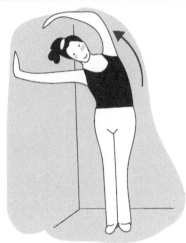

Stand at an arm's length away from the wall and place your right arm on it at shoulder height. Inhale and reach your left arm toward the wall, over your head. Return to the standing position.

Perform the movement dynamically (briskly, with energy) 15 times, then pause for 15 seconds. Repeat 3 times, then repeat on the other side.

Exercise 3

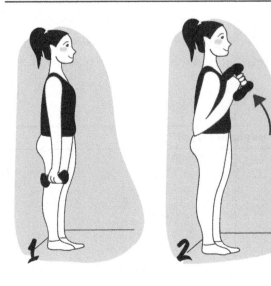

1.Use weights. Lean your body against the wall, with your glutes and abs contracted. Let your arms rest at your sides.

2.Flex your arms and bring the weights to your shoulders. Do not arch your back.

Perform the movement dynamically 15 times, then pause for 15 seconds. Repeat 3 times.

Exercise 4

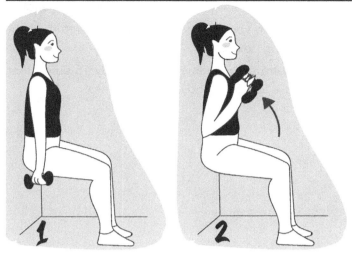

1. Use weights. Position yourself in the "chair position". Let your arms rest at your sides.

2. Inhale and flex your arms, bringing the weights to your shoulders. Exhale and extend the arms.

Perform the movement slowly 15 times, then pause for 15 seconds. Repeat 3 times.

Exercise 5

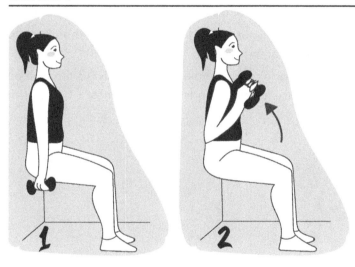

1. Use weights. Position yourself in the "chair position". Let your arms rest at your sides.

2. Flex your arms. Then extend the arms.

Perform the movement dynamically 15 times, then pause for 15 seconds. Repeat 3 times.

Exercise 6

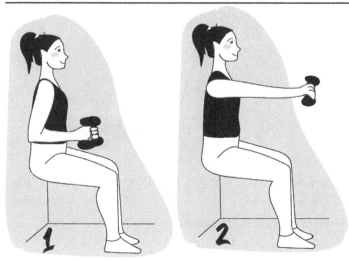

1. Use weights. Position yourself in the "chair position". Bend your elbows to a 90-degree angle.

2. Extend your arms in front of you at shoulder height and hold this position for 3 long breaths.

Perform the movement 15 times, then pause for 15 seconds. Repeat 3 times.

Exercise 7

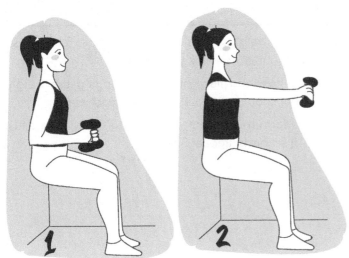

1. Use weights. Position yourself in the "chair position". Bend your elbows to a 90-degree angle.

2. Stretch your arms out in front, then return to the starting position.

Perform the movement dynamically 15 times, then pause for 15 seconds. Repeat 3 times.

Exercise 8

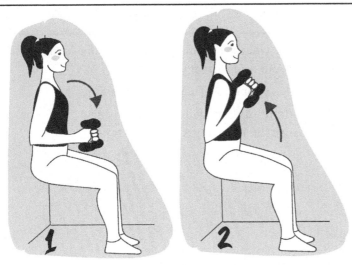

1. Use weights. Position yourself in the "chair position". Bend your elbows to a 90-degree angle.

2. Bring your hands to your chest and then back to the starting position.

Perform the movement dynamically 15 times, then pause for 15 seconds. Repeat 3 times.

Exercise 9

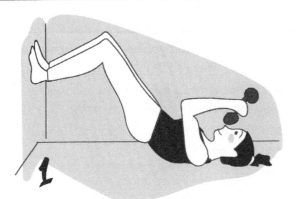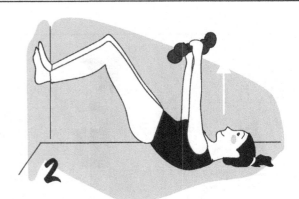

1. Keeping your feet firm against the wall, get into the bridge position. Use weights. Exhale and bend your elbows so the weights are to your forehead.

2. Inhale and extend arms to the ceiling without coming down from the bridge position.

Perform the movement slowly 15 times, then pause for 15 seconds. Repeat 3 times.

Exercise 10

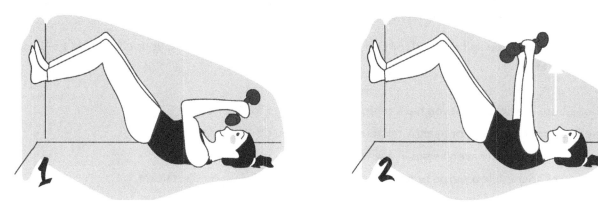

1. Keeping your feet firm against the wall, get into the bridge position. Use weights. Bend your elbows so the weights are close to your forehead.

2. Then extend your arms to the ceiling without coming down from the bridge position.

Perform the movement dynamically 15 times, then pause for 15 seconds. Repeat 3 times.

Final relaxation

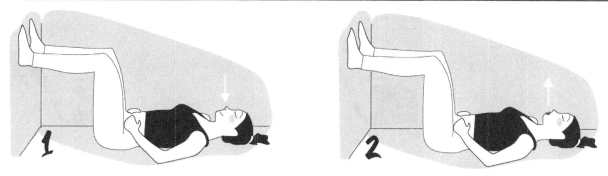

1. Place your feet on the wall and rest your hands on your belly. Keep your eyes closed. Breathe in slowly through your nose until you feel your belly rise under your hands.

2. Exhale slowly with your mouth ajar, relaxing the muscles in your face. Repeat for 2 minutes.

Tip of the Day: The slimming power of good deeds

Why does offering support to others have a positive influence on staying fit and losing weight? Simple: Those who give kindness generate a desire in others to give back. (If you meet people who are not infected by kindness, push them away!) Being kind to colleagues, friends, and family creates an environment of overall well-being that is supportive and will encourage you to maintain healthy behaviors and healthy food choices.

Doing good generates well-being and kindness!

PAUSE DAY 14: 5 ideas for rewarding things to do

Never forget to be kind to yourself first and foremost. Here are 5 ideas for rewarding your efforts and the beautiful person you are:

- Borrow a book from the library that you have been wanting to read for a long time.
- Treat yourself to a special dinner or healthy takeout meal that you don't have to cook.
- Spend time with a friend you haven't seen in a while.
- Do you like movies? Schedule a movie or theater night. If you prefer, buy a concert ticket.
- Take time for a beauty treatment at a salon or at home with a face mask and a warm bath.

WORKOUT DAY 15

Exercise 1

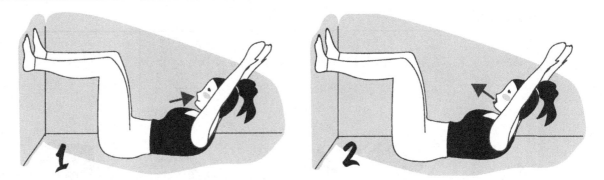

1. Keep your feet firmly against the wall, your arms close to your ears, and your shoulders raised off the ground. Inhale deeply and slowly through your nose.
2. Slowly exhale through your mouth, holding the position.

Perform the movement following the breath 15 times, then pause for 15 seconds. Repeat 3 times.

Exercise 2

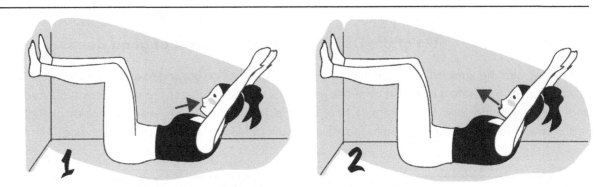

1. Keep your feet firmly against the wall, arms close to your ears, and shoulders raised off the ground; quickly inhale through your nose.
2. Slowly exhale through your mouth, holding the position.

Perform the movement dynamically (briskly, with energy) 15 times, then pause for 15 seconds. Repeat 3 times.

Exercise 3

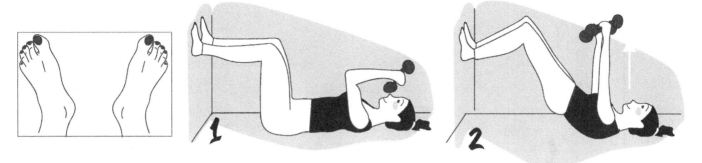

1. Rest your feet against the wall, slightly apart. Keep your gaze upward. Using weights, bend your arms close to your forehead.

2. Then extend your arms to the ceiling and go into the bridge position.

Perform the movement dynamically 15 times, then pause for 15 seconds. Repeat 3 times.

Exercise 4

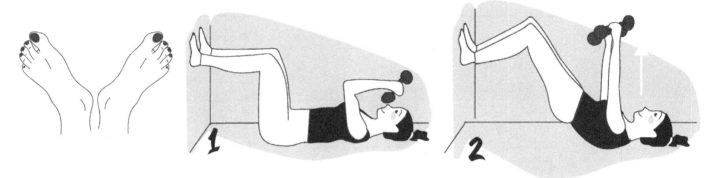

1. Rest your feet against the wall, toes facing out. Keep your gaze upward. Using weights, inhale and bend your elbows so your hands are close to your forehead.

2. Then exhale, extend arms to the ceiling and go into the bridge position.

Perform the movement slowly following the breath 15 times, then pause for 15 seconds. Repeat 3 times.

Exercise 5

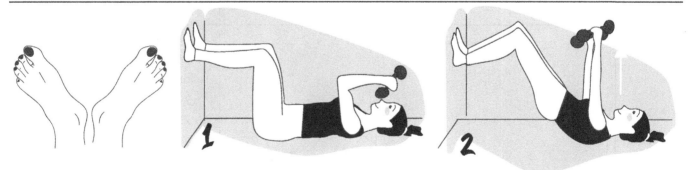

1. Rest your feet against the wall, toes open. Keep your gaze upward. Using weights, bend your elbows so your hands are close to your forehead.

2. Then extend arms to the ceiling and go into the bridge position.

Perform the movement dynamically 15 times, then pause for 15 seconds. Repeat 3 times.

Exercise 6

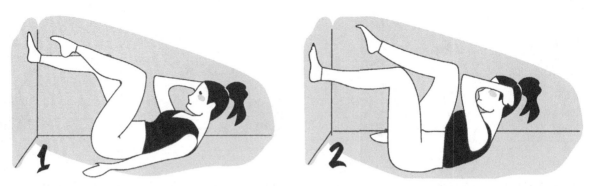

1. Keep your right foot firmly against the wall. Exhale and bring your right elbow close to your left knee. Inhale and bring the foot back against the wall.

2. Exhale and bring your left elbow close to your right knee. Inhale and return the foot to the wall.

Perform the movement slowly 15 times, then pause for 15 seconds. Repeat 3 times.

Exercise 7

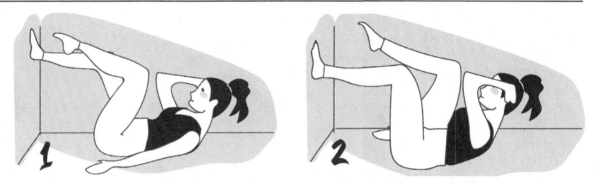

1. Keep your right foot firmly against the wall. Bring your right elbow close to your left knee.

2. Then switch sides.

Perform the movement dynamically 15 times, then pause for 15 seconds. Repeat 3 times.

Exercise 8

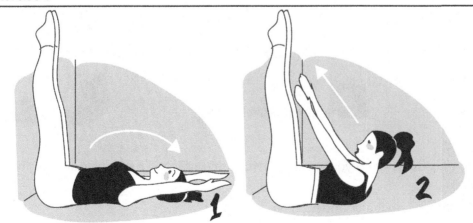

1. Rest your outstretched legs against the wall, your back flat on the floor. Inhale and bring your arms over your head.

2. Exhale and extend your arms toward your toes, lifting your shoulders off the ground.

Perform the movement slowly 15 times, then pause for 15 seconds. Repeat 3 times.

Exercise 9

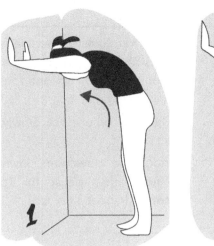

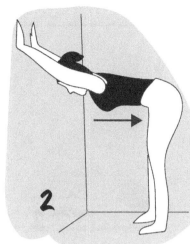

1. Lean your hands against the wall and push against the wall, hunching your back.

2. Return your back to a horizontal position.

Perform the movement dynamically 15 times, then pause for 15 seconds. Repeat 3 times.

Exercise 10

1. Lean your hands against the wall and push against the wall, hunching your back. Hold the position for three long breaths.

2. Return your back to a horizontal position and take three long breaths.

Perform the movement slowly 15 times, then pause for 15 seconds. Repeat 3 times.

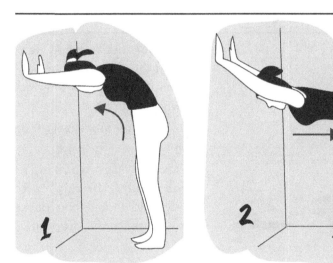

Tip of the Day: How to renew motivation

You are halfway through your challenge. You may be feeling tired and unmotivated because you are not yet seeing the results you hope for. Follow these simple tips to move forward, more motivated and determined than before:

• Accept that you will have moments of hesitation – you are human!

• Think back to the initial motivation that prompted you to undertake the challenge.

• Focus on the goals and benefits you will have once you reach the finish line.

• Reread the progress you made and marked in your personal journal.

• Remember that you started from scratch and look at where you are now!

Having difficult days is normal!

Exercise 1

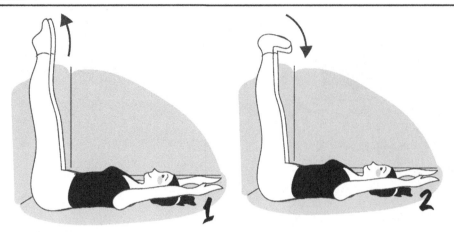

1. Rest your outstretched legs against the wall and your back flat on the floor. Flex one foot slowly, then point it.

2. Flex the other foot slowly, then point it.

Perform the movement slowly 15 times, then pause for 15 seconds. Repeat 3 times.

Exercise 2

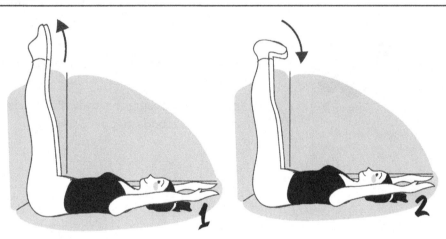

Rest your outstretched legs against the wall and your back flat on the floor. Flex one foot slowly, then point it.

Flex the other foot slowly, then point it.

Perform the movement dynamically (briskly, with energy) 15 times, then pause for 15 seconds. Repeat 3 times.

Exercise 3

1. Keep your legs straight against the wall and your arms stretched back over your head.

2. Bend your legs toward your right side. Contract your glutes and abs and maintain your gaze upward. Hold the position for 3 slow breaths.

Pause for 15 seconds and repeat the exercise on the other side. Repeat 3 times.

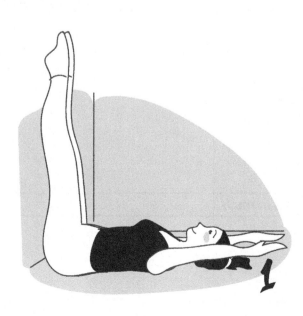

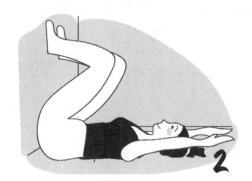

Exercise 4

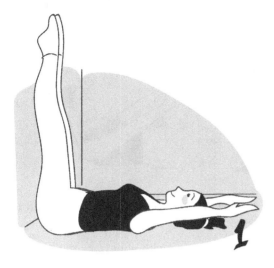

1. Keep your outstretched legs against the wall and your arms stretched back over your head.

2. Bend your legs toward your right side. Then extend your legs and bend them toward your left side. Do not arch the back.

Perform the movement dynamically 15 times, then pause for 15 seconds. Repeat 3 times.

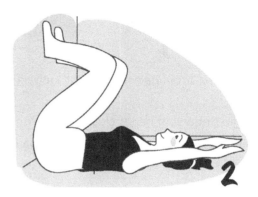

Exercise 5

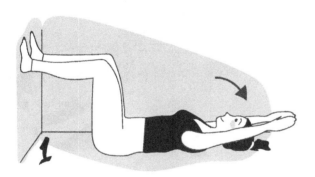
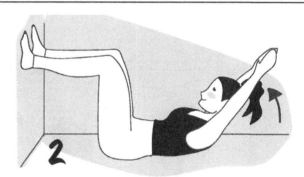

1. Keep your feet firm against the wall. Contract your abdominals. Inhale and bring your arms outstretched over your head.

2. Exhale and lift your arms and shoulders off the floor. Take three long breaths and return with your back to the floor.

Perform the movement slowly 15 times, then pause for 15 seconds. Repeat 3 times.

Exercise 6

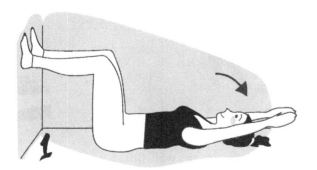
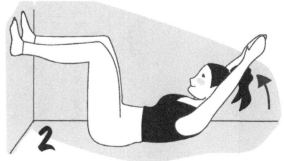

1. Keep your feet firm against the wall. Contract your abdominals. Bring your arms outstretched over your head.

2. Lift your arms and shoulders off the floor. Then return your back to the floor.

Perform the movement dynamically 15 times, then pause for 15 seconds. Repeat 3 times.

Exercise 7

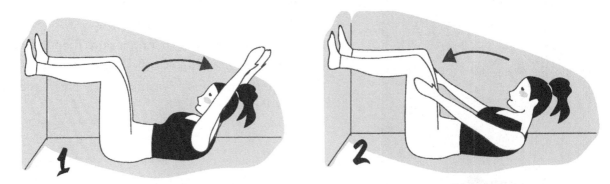

1. Keep your feet firm against the wall. Contract your abdominals. Inhale and lift your arms and shoulders off the floor.

2. Exhale and bring your hands close to your knees. Take three long breaths and return with your back to the floor.

Perform the movement slowly 15 times, then pause for 15 seconds. Repeat 3 times.

Exercise 8

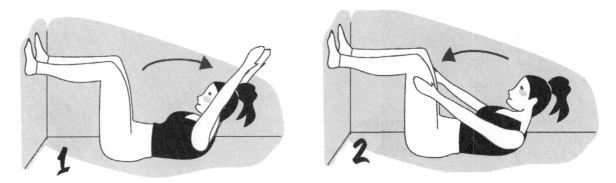

1. Keep your feet firm against the wall. Contract your abdominals. Lift your arms and shoulders off the floor.

2. Bring your hands close to your knees, then bring your arms over your head.

Perform the movement dynamically 15 times, then pause for 15 seconds. Repeat 3 times.

Exercise 9

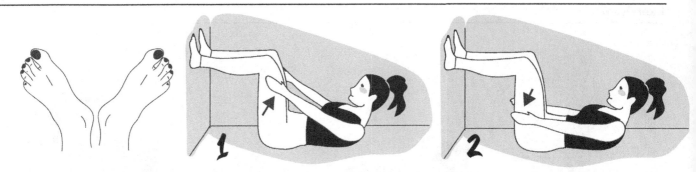

1. Rest your feet against the wall, toes facing out. Keep your gaze toward the wall. Bring your hands to your knees.

2. Then bring your hands close to the floor.

Move your arms up and down dynamically 15 times, then pause for 15 seconds. Repeat 3 times.

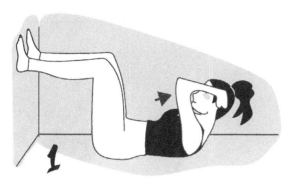 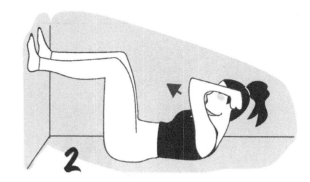

1. Keep your feet firm against the wall. Contract your abdominals. Lift your shoulders off the floor. Place your hands behind your head. Inhale deeply through your nose.
2. Exhale deeply through the mouth.

Perform the movement slowly 15 times, then pause for 15 seconds. Repeat 3 times.

Final relaxation

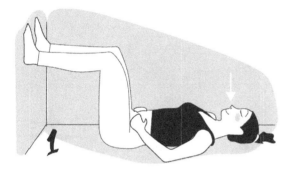 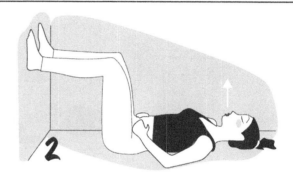

1. Place your feet on the wall and rest your hands on your belly. Keep your eyes closed. Breathe in slowly through your nose until you feel your belly rise under your hands.
2. Exhale slowly with your mouth ajar and relax the muscles in your face. Repeat for 2 minutes.

Tip of the Day: Sleep and wellness

Why does sleep help you lose weight and stay fit?

Because people tend to crave more sugary and fatty foods when they are tired, looking for quick sources of energy to compensate for the lack of rest.

In addition, sleep affects metabolism. A lack of sleep can slow down your metabolism and reduce your body's ability to burn calories.

Sleep is good for you, and taking care of your sleep is a great way to take care of your fitness!

WORKOUT DAY 17

Exercise 1

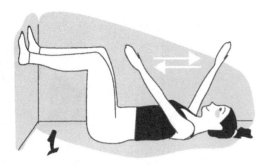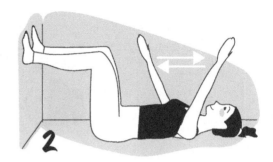

1. Keep your gaze upward and your feet firm against the wall. Raise your outstretched arms, one angled down and one angled up, with your shoulders resting firmly on the floor.

2. Alternate the positions of your arms by moving them forward and backward energetically.

Perform the movement 15 times, then pause for 15 seconds. Repeat 3 times.

Exercise 2

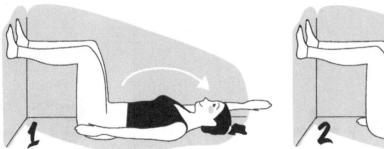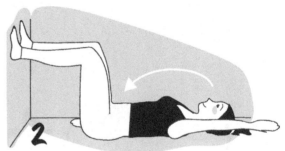

1. Keep your gaze upward and your feet firm against the wall. Exhale and straighten your arms, one by your head and one by your side, and contract your abs.

2. Inhale and alternate your arms slowly, following the breath.

Perform the movement following the breath 15 times, then pause for 15 seconds. Repeat 3 times.

Exercise 3

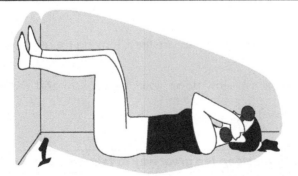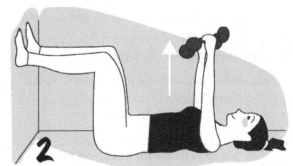

1. Use weights. Keep your gaze upward and your feet firm against the wall. Exhale and bend your arms so your hands are close to your ears.

2. Inhale and extend your arms slowly.

Perform the movement following the breath 15 times, then pause for 15 seconds. Repeat 3 times.

Exercise 4

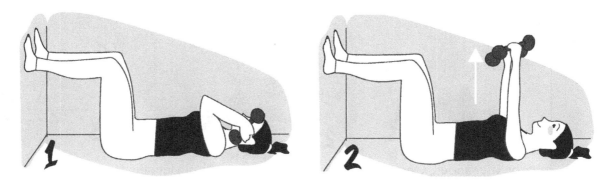

1. Use weights. Keep your gaze upward and your feet firm against the wall. Bend your arms so your hands are close to your ears.

2. Then extend your arms.

Perform the movement dynamically (briskly, with energy) 15 times, then pause for 15 seconds. Repeat 3 times.

Exercise 5

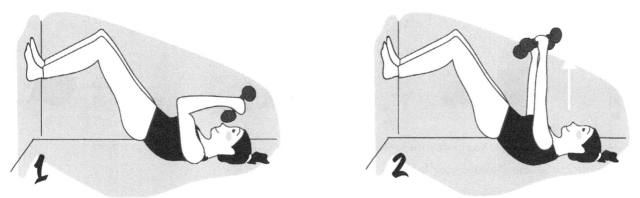

1. With your feet firm against the wall, get into the bridge position. Use weights. Exhale and keep your arms flexed close to your forehead.

2. Inhale and extend your arms without coming down from the bridge position.

Perform the movement slowly 15 times, then pause for 15 seconds. Repeat 3 times.

Exercise 6

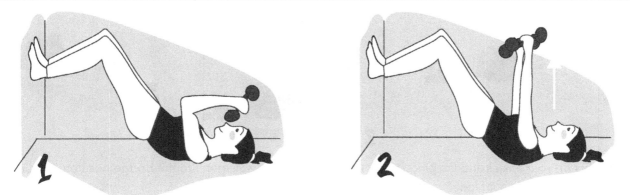

1. With your feet firm against the wall, get into the bridge position. Use weights. Keep your arms flexed close to your forehead.

2. Then extend your arms without coming down from the bridge position.

Perform the movement dynamically 15 times, then pause for 15 seconds. Repeat 3 times.

Exercise 7

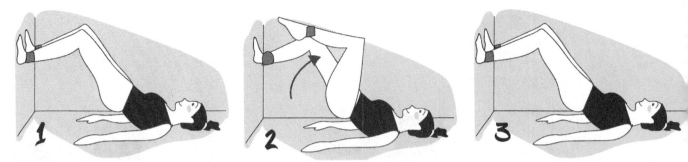

1. Place weights on your ankles. Keeping your feet firm against the wall, get into the bridge position.

2. Exhale and bring one knee toward your face.

3. Inhale and return to the bridge position.

Perform the movement slowly 15 times, then pause for 15 seconds. Repeat 3 times, then switch sides.

Exercise 8

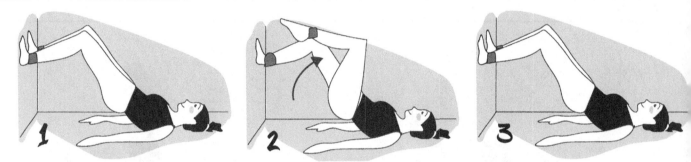

1. Place weights on your ankles. Keeping your feet firm against the wall, get into the bridge position.

2. Exhale and bring one knee toward your face.

3. Inhale and return to the bridge position.

Perform the movement dynamically 15 times, then pause for 15 seconds. Repeat 3 times, then switch sides.

Exercise 9

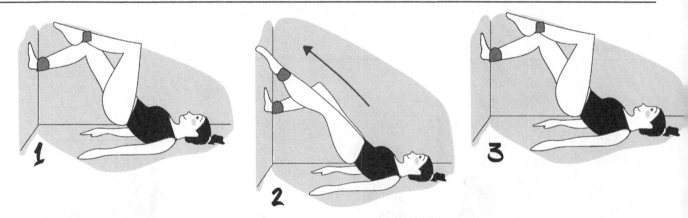

1. With weights on your ankles and keeping your feet firm against the wall, get into the bridge position. Exhale and bring one knee toward your face.

2. Inhale and extend that leg.

3. Exhale and bring the knee back toward your face.

Perform the movement slowly 15 times, then pause for 15 seconds. Repeat 3 times, then switch sides.

Exercise 10

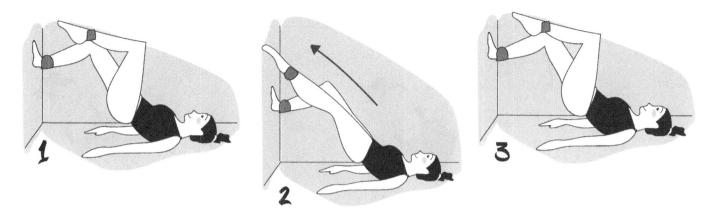

1. With weights on your ankles and keeping your feet firm against the wall, get into the bridge position. Exhale and bring one knee toward your face.
2. Inhale and extend that leg.
3. Exhale and bring the knee back toward your face.

Perform the movement dynamically 15 times, then pause for 15 seconds. Repeat 3 times, then switch sides.

Final relaxation

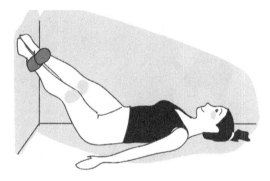

Rest your feet on the wall and keep your arms along your sides. Bring your knees to the right and take 3 long breaths.

Bring your knees to the left and take 3 long breaths. Repeat for 2 minutes.

Tip of the Day: The power of smoothies

Fruit and vegetable concentrates are an excellent source of nutrients. They are easy to prepare and contribute to better digestion and a feeling of fullness. My favorite? Apple, carrot, celery and ginger!

Try replacing a snack or meal with a smoothie!

WORKOUT DAY 18

Exercise 1

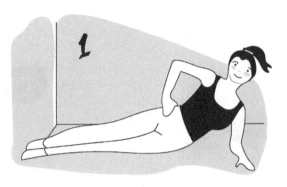 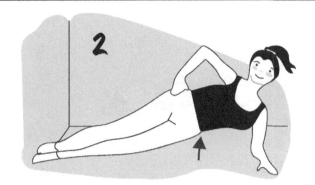

1. Lie on your side, with your weight on your arm on the ground. Keep your other arm resting on your side.

2. Lift your hip and hold the position for three long breaths.

Perform the movement slowly 15 times, then pause for 15 seconds. Repeat on the opposite side.

Exercise 2

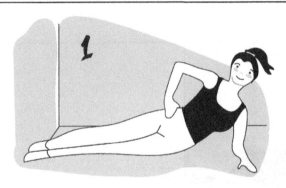 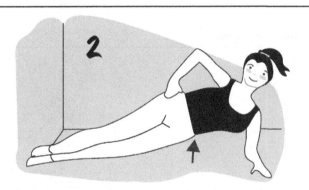

1. Lie on your side, with your weight on your arm on the ground. Keep your other arm resting on your side.

2. Lift your hip and then return to the starting position.

Perform the movement dynamically (briskly, with energy) 15 times, then pause for 15 seconds. Repeat on the opposite side.

Exercise 3

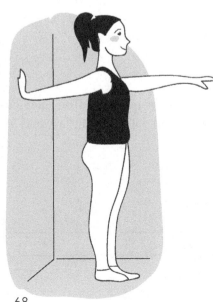

1. Standing in front of the wall, bring one arm forward and one arm behind you. Rest your hand against the wall to stretch the shoulder joint.

2. Hold the position for 3 slow breaths.

Pause for 15 seconds and repeat the exercise with the other arm. Repeat 3 times.

Exercise 4

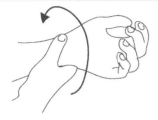

Pause and loosen both wrists before continuing.

Rotate your wrists in a twisting motion to the right and left.

Perform a gentle massage.

Exercise 5

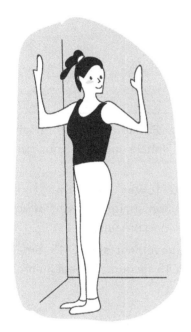

Standing in front of the wall, place one forearm against the wall and rotate your upper body in the opposite direction to stretch the joint.

Hold the position for 3 slow breaths.

Pause for 15 seconds and repeat the exercise with the other arm. Repeat 3 times.

Exercise 6

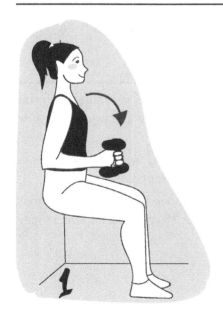
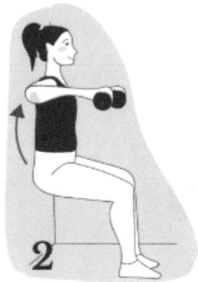

1.Use weights. Position yourself in the "chair position". Exhale and bend your arms at a right angle so your hands are above your thighs.

2.Inhale and lift the elbows to a horizontal position.

Perform the movement slowly 15 times, then pause for 15 seconds. Repeat 3 times.

Exercise 7

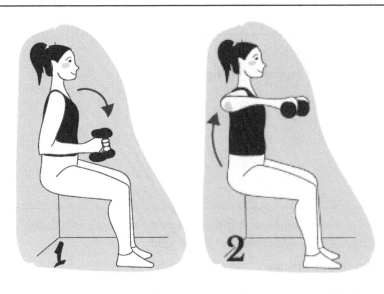

1. Use weights. Position yourself in the "chair position". Bend your arms at a right angle so your hands are above your knees.

2. Lift the elbows to a horizontal position.

Perform the movement dynamically 15 times, then pause for 15 seconds. Repeat 3 times.

Exercise 8

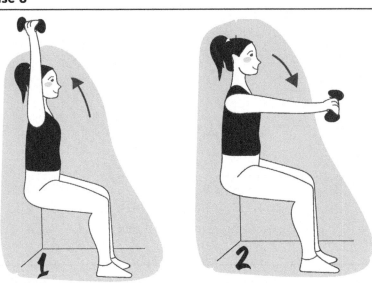

1. Use weights. Position yourself in the 'chair position'. Inhale and raise your arms overhead.

2. Exhale and lower the arms to a horizontal position straight in front of you and take three long breaths.

Perform the movement slowly 15 times, then pause for 15 seconds. Repeat 3 times.

Exercise 8

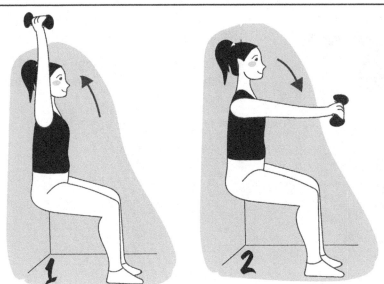

1. Use weights. Position yourself in the "chair position". Inhale and bring your arms overhead.

2. Exhale and bring arms to a horizontal position at shoulder height.

Perform the movement slowly 15 times, then pause for 15 seconds. Repeat 3 times.

Exercise 9

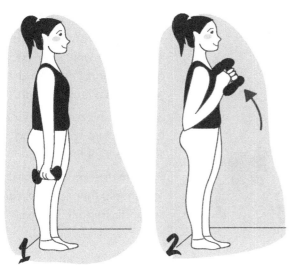

1. Use weights. Lean against the wall with your glutes and abs contracted. Let your arms rest at your sides.

2. Bend your elbows, bringing the weights to the front of your shoulders. Do not arch your back.

Perform the movement dynamically 15 times, then pause for 15 seconds. Repeat 3 times.

Final relaxation

Sitting on the floor with legs crossed, extend one arm toward the opposite shoulder, grasp the elbow, and gently pull the arm toward the torso. Hold the position for 1 minute and then repeat, changing sides.

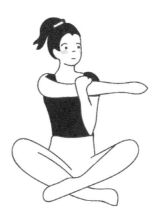

Tip of the Day: Herbal teas for every need

Whatever your mild ailment, nature comes to the rescue with infusions and herbal teas. Any natural-goods shop in your town can recommend herbal combinations specific to your needs, but you can also rely on the well-stocked supermarket shelves to get you started. Here are a few teas and their remedies: Chamomile for sleep. Valerian for relaxing and coping with stress. Fennel for deflating the belly. Ginger for digestion. Lemon balm to fight colds. Licorice for constipation. These are just examples of what you can choose to stay in shape easily and naturally.

Nature is your ally!

WORKOUT DAY 19

Exercise 1

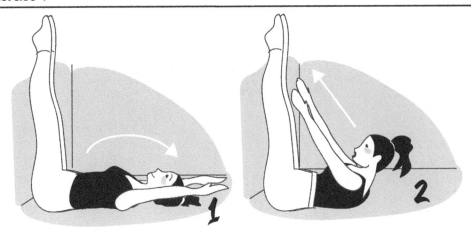

1.Rest your outstretched legs against the wall, your back flat on the floor. Inhale and bring your arms over your head.

2.Exhale and extend your arms toward your toes, lifting your shoulders off the floor.

Perform the movement slowly 15 times, then pause for 15 seconds. Repeat 3 times.

Exercise 2

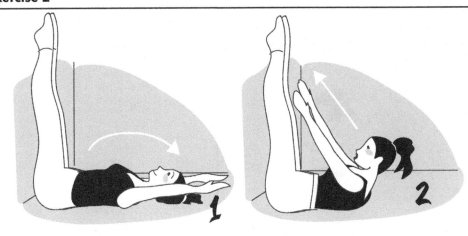

1.Rest your outstretched legs against the wall, your back flat on the floor. Bring your arms over your head.

2.Then extend your arms toward your toes, lifting your shoulders off the floor.

Perform the movement dynamically (briskly, with energy) 15 times, then pause for 15 seconds. Repeat 3 times.

Exercise 3

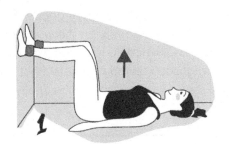 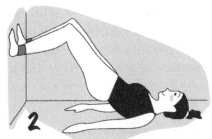 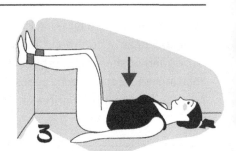

1. Use ankle weights. Position yourself with your feet on the wall and your arms along your sides.

2. Lift your glutes into the bridge position, keeping your gaze upward. Take three long breaths.

3. Return your glutes to the floor.

Perform the movement slowly 15 times, then pause for 15 seconds. Repeat 3 times.

Exercise 4

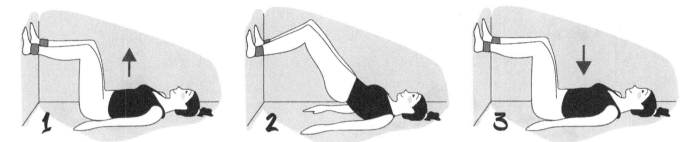

1. Use ankle weights. Position yourself with your feet on the wall and your arms along your sides.

2. Lift your glutes into the bridge position, keeping your gaze upward.

3. Return your glutes to the floor.

Perform the movement dynamically 15 times, then pause for 15 seconds. Repeat 3 times.

Exercise 5

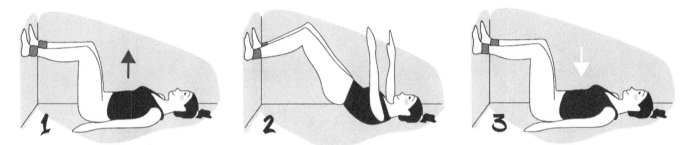

1. Use ankle weights. Position yourself with your feet on the wall and your arms along your sides.

2. Lift your buttocks into the bridge position with arms stretched toward the ceiling. Keep your gaze upward. Take three long breaths.

3. Return your glutes and arms to the floor.

Perform the movement slowly 15 times, then pause for 15 seconds. Repeat 3 times.

Exercise 6

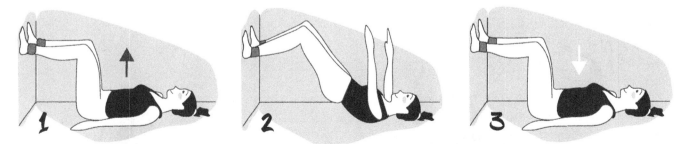

1. Use ankle weights. Position yourself with your feet on the wall and your arms along your sides.

2. Lift your buttocks into the bridge position with arms extended toward the ceiling. Keep your gaze upward.

3. Return your glutes and arms to the floor.

Perform the movement dynamically 15 times, then pause for 15 seconds. Repeat 3 times.

Exercise 7

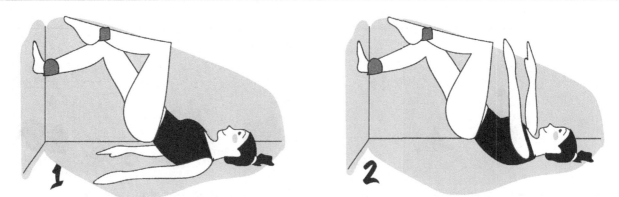

1. Use ankle weights. Position yourself with your feet on the wall and your arms along your sides. Lift one knee toward your head and take three long breaths.

2. Raise your arms toward the ceiling and take three long breaths. Keep your gaze upward, then return to the starting position.

Perform the movement slowly 15 times, then pause for 15 seconds. Repeat 3 times with both legs.

Exercise 8

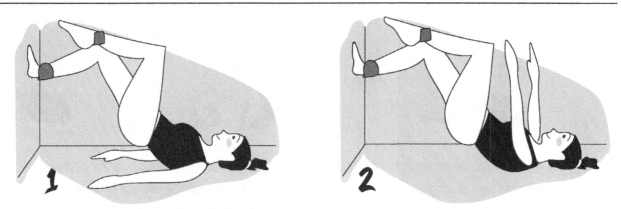

1. Use ankle weights. Position yourself with your feet on the wall and your arms along your sides. Lift one knee toward your head.

2. Raise your arms toward the ceiling, then return the arms to the floor and your foot to the wall.

Perform the movement dynamically 15 times, then pause for 15 seconds. Repeat 3 times with both legs.

Exercise 9

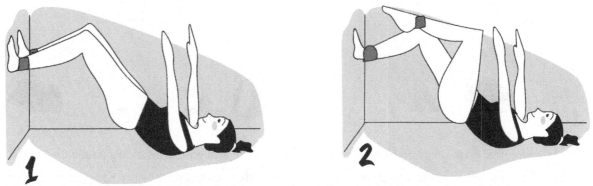

1. Use ankle weights. Position yourself with your feet against the wall and arms stretched overhead.

2. Bend one leg toward your head and take three long breaths. Keep your gaze upward.

Return your foot to the wall. Perform the movement slowly 15 times, then pause for 15 seconds. Repeat 3 times with both legs.

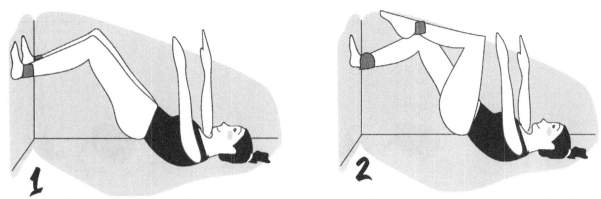

1. Use ankle weights. Position yourself with your feet against the wall and arms stretched overhead. Lift your hips into the bridge position.

2. Bend one leg toward your head, then return your foot to the wall.

Perform the movement dynamically 15 times, then pause for 15 seconds. Repeat 3 times with both legs.

Final relaxation

Stand in front of the wall and lean against it on your hands. Flex one foot against the wall and straighten the knee to stretch the Achilles tendon and calf muscles. Hold the position for 1 minute and then repeat with the other leg.

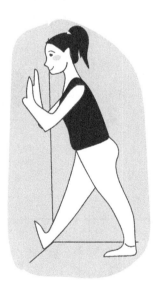

Tip of the Day: Watchword: Dare!

An ancient proverb says, "If you ask, you will be ignorant for 5 minutes; if you don't ask, you will be ignorant all your life!"

What does this proverb teach us? That it doesn't matter if you appear clumsy, awkward or incompetent in a given context or at a given time. What matters is be daring so that you can improve yourself. Dare to ask. Dare to do. Dare to exist!

Daring means giving yourself a chance to improve!

WORKOUT DAY 20

Exercise 1

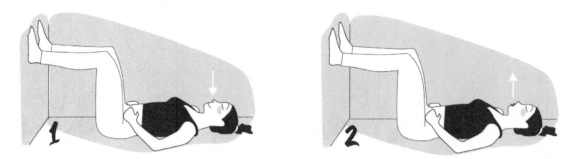

1. Place your feet on the wall with your hands resting on your belly. Keep your eyes closed. Breathe in slowly through your nose until you feel your belly rise under your hands.

2. Exhale slowly with your mouth ajar and relax the muscles in your face. Repeat for 2 minutes.

Exercise 2

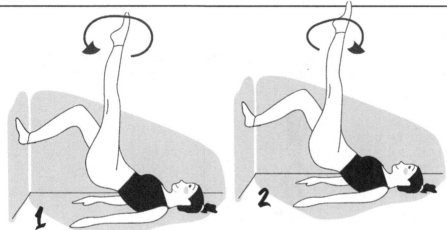

1. With one foot against the wall, lift your pelvis off the ground. Lift your other leg straight to the ceiling and slowly rotate clockwise 15 times.

2. With the same leg, slowly rotate counterclockwise 15 times.

Perform the movement slowly with both legs, then pause for 15 seconds. Repeat 3 times.

Exercise 3

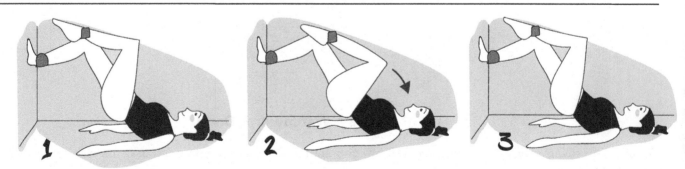

1. Use ankle weights. Place one foot on the wall and bend the other leg toward the ceiling. Keep your arms along your sides.

2. Bring your knee close to your forehead and take three long breaths.

3. Return your foot close to the wall.

Perform the movement slowly 15 times, then pause for 15 seconds. Repeat 3 times with both legs.

Exercise 4

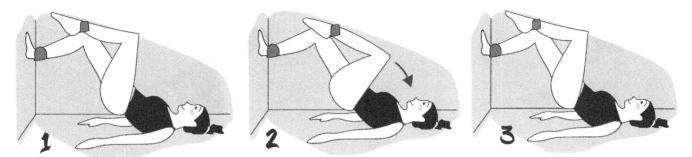

1. Use ankle weights. Place one foot on the wall and bend the other knee toward the ceiling. Keep your arms along your sides.

2. Bring your knee closer to your forehead.

3. Then return with your foot close to the wall.

Perform the movement dynamically 15 times, then pause for 15 seconds. Repeat 3 times with both legs.

Exercise 5

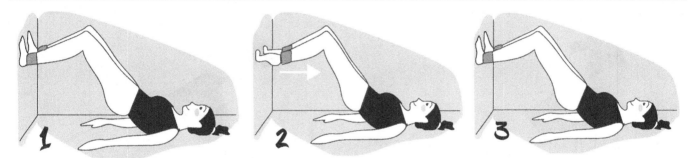

1. Use ankle weights. Position yourself with your feet against the wall, keeping your arms at your sides.

2. Lift your heels and contract your glutes. Take three long breaths.

3. Return your heels to the wall.

Perform the movement slowly 15 times, then pause for 15 seconds. Repeat 3 times.

Exercise 6

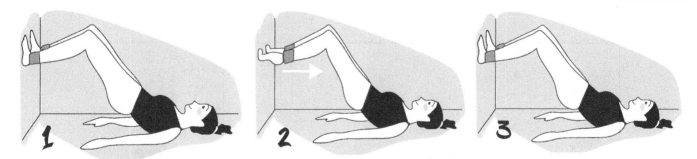

1.Use ankle weights. Position yourself with your feet against the wall, keeping your arms at your sides.

2. Lift your heels and contract your glutes.

3. Return your heels to the wall.

Perform the movement dynamically 15 times, then pause for 15 seconds. Repeat 3 times.

Exercise 7

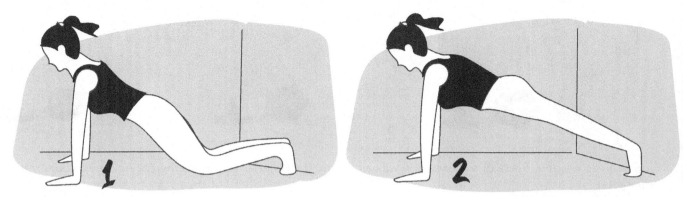

1. Get in a push-up position with your feet against the wall and your hands on the floor. Keep your legs bent, knees resting on the floor.

2. Straighten your legs and hold the position for 3 long breaths.

Perform the movement slowly 15 times, then pause for 15 seconds. Repeat 3 times.

Exercise 8

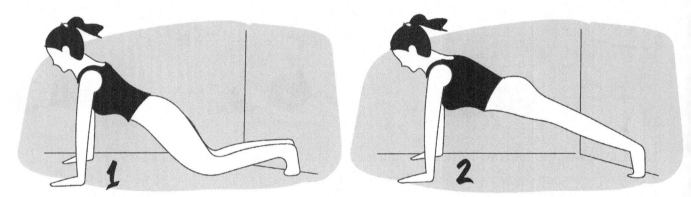

1. Get in a push-up position with your feet against the wall and your hands on the floor. Keep your legs bent, knees resting on the floor.

2. Straighten your legs, keeping your back straight.

Perform the movement dynamically 15 times, then pause for 15 seconds. Repeat 3 times.

Exercise 9

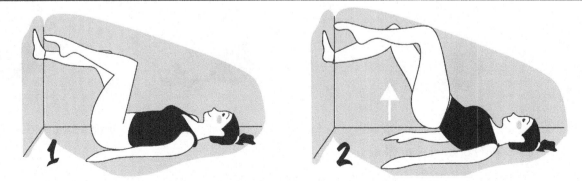

1. Rest your feet on the wall with your hands along your sides. Inhale and move one foot away from the wall.

2. Exhale and lift the buttocks. Hold the position for 3 long breaths.

Perform the movement slowly 15 times, then pause for 15 seconds. Repeat 3 times with both legs.

Exercise 10

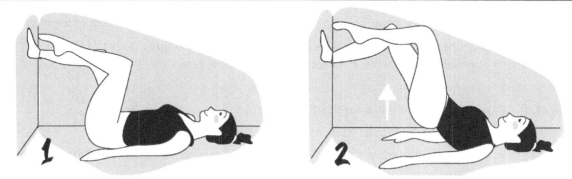

1. Rest your feet on the wall and keep your hands along your sides. Move one foot away from the wall.

2. Lift the buttocks. Then return to the starting position.

Perform the movement dynamically 15 times, then pause for 15 seconds. Repeat 3 times with both legs.

Final relaxation

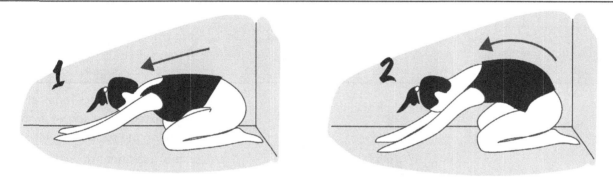

1. Sit on your heels and stretch your arms out in front of you. Take three long breaths.

2. Round your back and take three long breaths.

Perform the movement slowly 15 times, then pause for 15 seconds. Repeat 3 times.

Tip of the Day: Do you have to give up dessert?

It is well known that reducing sugar consumption is helpful in losing weight, but is it really necessary to give up all sweet things completely? The answer is no! There are naturally sweet alternatives that offer health benefits without contributing to weight gain; here are some ideas: Use fresh fruits such as strawberries, apples, blueberries, and citrus fruits to benefit from their natural sweetness provided by fructose. Fruit is rich in fiber, vitamins and antioxidants, which promote satiety and overall health. Honey is a natural sweetener with a high antioxidant content. In addition, honey is sweeter than sugar, so you need less of it to get the same sweet taste. Stevia is a natural sweetener extracted from sugarcane leaves. It is sweet but contains no calories, so it can be an alternative for those looking for a sugar substitute.

Use your imagination to search for sweet foods that are not fattening!

PAUSE DAY 21: Getting familiar with the new routine

Congratulations! You have made it to the third week of your Pilates to the Wall challenge. This is a great milestone and you are only one week away from completing the challenge. As you finish the challenge, it is important to continue to keep yourself in shape with daily workouts and a healthy diet to make the most of these workouts.

During this off day, I recommend that you take note of the things you are enjoying and what you can turn around instead. Answer these questions and use the answers to formulate new goals.

- What time of day allows you to feel most energized and focused during your workouts?
- Do you need support from family or friends to maintain a workout habit?
- Which exercises have given you the most satisfaction and gratification so far? Memorize them to repeat them in the future.
- Have you had difficulty maintaining consistency in training because of work or personal commitments? What can help you with this?
- What changes in your daily habits support your commitment to regular training?
- Have you found that working out has helped you manage daily stress and improve your overall mood?
- Do you feel the need to intensify your physical activity to achieve your goals or do you need to reduce the intensity to avoid overtraining?

WORKOUT DAY 22

Exercise 1

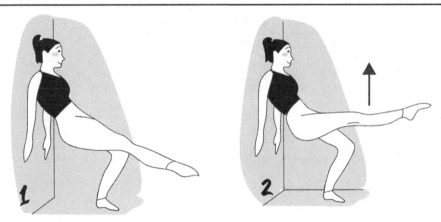

1.Lean your shoulders against the wall and extend one leg in front of you, bending the supporting leg.

2.Lift the leg until it is just past horizontal and take three long breaths.

Perform the movement slowly 15 times, then pause for 15 seconds. Repeat 3 times with both legs.

Exercise 2

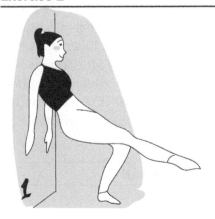
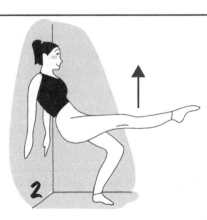

1.Lean your shoulders against the wall and extend one leg in front of you, bending the supporting leg.

2.Raise your leg just past horizontal and then return to the lower position.

Perform the movement dynamically 15 times, then pause for 15 seconds. Repeat 3 times with both legs.

Exercise 3

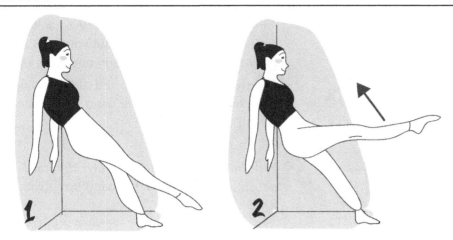

1. Lean your shoulders against the wall and extend one leg in front of you, keeping the supporting leg straight.

2. Lift the leg past horizontal and take three long breaths.

Perform the movement slowly 15 times, then pause for 15 seconds. Repeat 3 times with both legs.

Exercise 4

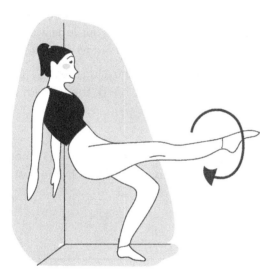

1. Lean your shoulders against the wall and extend one leg in front of you, keeping the supporting leg straight.

2. Slowly perform clockwise, circular movements with your foot 15 times, then pause for 15 seconds. Repeat 3 times with both legs.

3. Then slowly perform counterclockwise circular movements with your foot 15 times, then pause for 15 seconds. Repeat 3 times with both legs.

Exercise 5

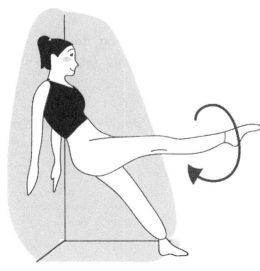

1. Lean your shoulders against the wall and extend one leg in front of you, keeping the supporting leg straight.

2. Slowly perform clockwise, circular movements with your foot 15 times, then pause for 15 seconds. Repeat 3 times with both legs.

3. Then slowly perform counterclockwise circular movements with your foot 15 times, then pause for 15 seconds. Repeat 3 times with both legs.

Exercise 6

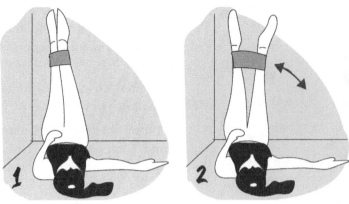

1.Place the elastic band around your ankles. Rest your back on the floor and put your legs against the wall. Stretch your right arm out to the side.

2.Move your right leg to the side, feeling the resistance from the rubber band. Take three long breaths.

Perform the movement slowly 15 times, then pause for 15 seconds. Repeat 3 times with both legs.

Exercise 7

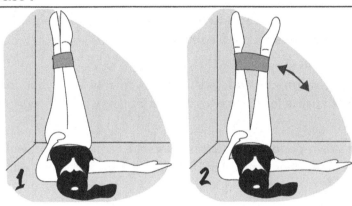

1.Place the elastic band around your ankles. Rest your back on the floor and put your legs against the wall. Stretch your right arm out to the side.

2.Move your right leg to the side, feeling the resistance from the rubber band, then return to the starting position.

Perform the movement dynamically 15 times, then pause for 15 seconds. Repeat 3 times with both legs.

Exercise 8

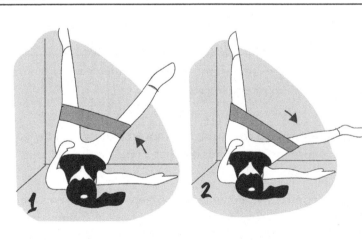

1.Place the elastic band around your thighs. Rest your back on the floor with your legs against the wall. Keep your right arm stretched out to the side.

2.Open your legs by pressing down on the rubber band with your right leg. Take three long breaths.

Perform the movement slowly 15 times, then pause for 15 seconds. Repeat 3 times with both legs.

Exercise 9

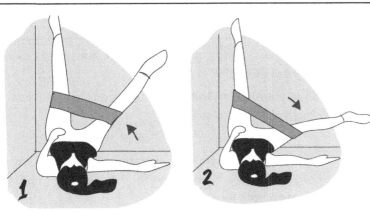

1. Place the elastic band around your thighs. Rest your back on the floor with your legs against the wall. Keep your right arm stretched out to the sides.

2. Open your legs by pressing down on the rubber band with your right leg. Then close.

Perform the movement dynamically 15 times, then pause for 15 seconds. Repeat 3 times with both legs.

Exercise 10

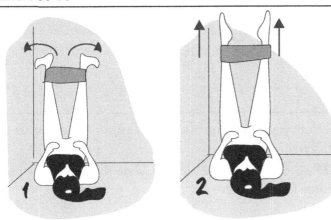

1. Put the elastic band around your ankles. Rest your back on the floor, legs against the wall. Flex your feet and press your legs apart while resisting against the rubber band.

2. Point your toes to the ceiling, then return your legs to the center.

Perform the movement slowly 15 times, then pause for 15 seconds. Repeat 3 times with both legs.

Final relaxation

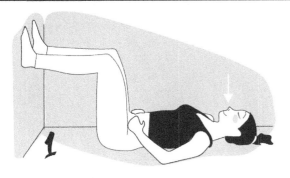 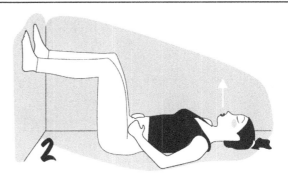

1. Place your feet on the wall, hands resting on your belly. Keep your eyes closed. Breathe in slowly through your nose until you feel your belly rise under your hands.

2. Exhale slowly with your mouth ajar and relax the muscles in your face. Repeat for 2 minutes.

Tip of the Day: Pizza – yes or no?

Pizza is a yes! Pizza is a healthy food if made in the traditional way, with quality products, such as fresh tomatoes and olive oil. If you have cravings for pizza but fear you'll have to give it up to lose weight, you're wrong. A small pizza marinara made with whole-wheat flour, tomato, garlic and a drizzle of olive oil is a complete, low-calorie meal. It is important not to drink carbonated beverages along with the pizza, and avoid adding toppings such as cheese, ham, sausage and salami. Opt for grilled vegetables or mushrooms instead!

All foods can be revisited and adapted to your needs.

WORKOUT DAY 23

Exercise 1

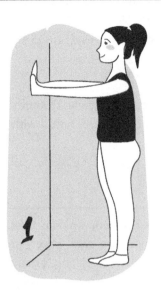 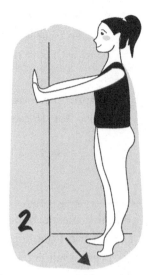

1.Place your hands on the wall for support, looking straight at the wall.

2.Slide your left leg to the side until your heel leaves the floor, then return to standing.

Perform the movement dynamically (briskly, with energy) 15 times, then pause for 15 seconds. Repeat 3 times with both legs.

Exercise 2

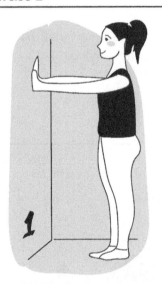 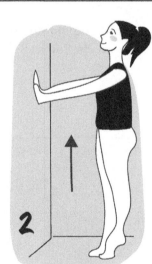

1.With your hands on the wall, stand straight and gaze at the wall.

2.Rise onto your toes and lift your gaze upward. Take three long breaths.

Perform the movement slowly 15 times, then pause for 15 seconds. Repeat 3 times.

Exercise 3

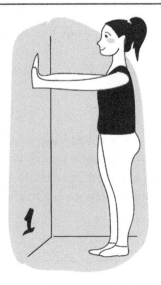 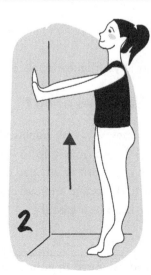

1.With your hands against the wall, stand straight and gaze at the wall.

2.Rise onto your toes and lift your gaze upward. Then return your heels to the floor.

Perform the movement dynamically 15 times, then pause for 15 seconds. Repeat 3 times.

Exercise 4

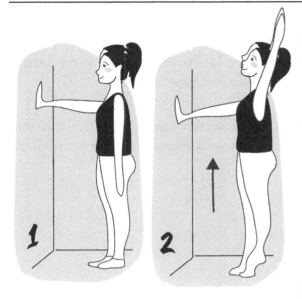

1. Place one hand on the wall with the other arm by your side.
2. Rise onto your toes and lift your arm overhead. Take three deep breaths.

Perform the movement slowly 15 times, then pause for 15 seconds. Repeat 3 times with both arms.

Exercise 5

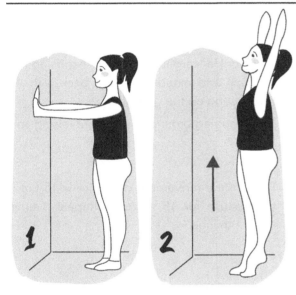

1. Lean your hands against the wall.
2. Rise onto your toes, then lift both arms overhead. Take three long breaths.

Perform the movement slowly 15 times, then pause for 15 seconds. Repeat 3 times.

Exercise 6

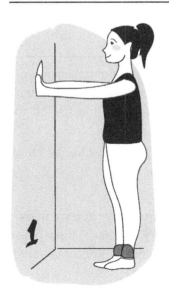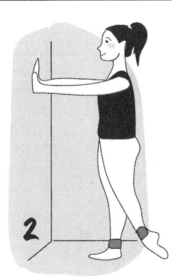

1. Use ankle weights. Lean your hands against the wall.
2. Extend your left foot behind you, toe to the ground. Then bring your feet together again.

Perform the movement dynamically 15 times, then pause for 15 seconds. Repeat 3 times with both legs.

Exercise 7

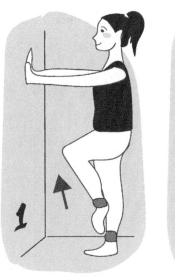 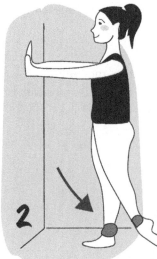

1. Use ankle weights. Lean your hands against the wall and lift your left knee.

2. Place your left foot behind you, toe to the ground. Then bring your feet together again.

Perform the movement dynamically 15 times, then pause for 15 seconds. Repeat 3 times with both legs.

Exercise 8

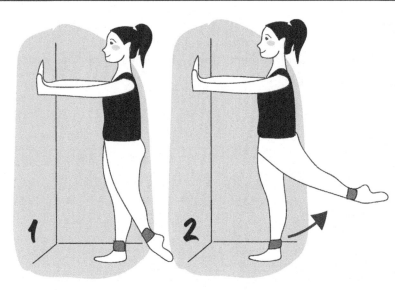

1. Use ankle weights. Lean your hands against the wall and extend one leg back with the toes resting on the ground.

2. Lift your leg behind you without raising your hips.

Perform the movement dynamically 15 times, then pause for 15 seconds. Repeat 3 times with both legs.

Exercise 8

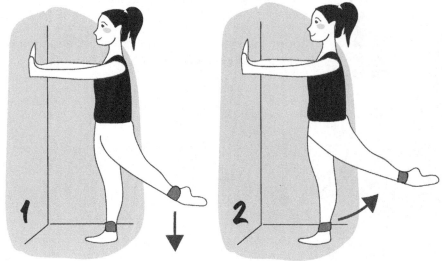

1. Use ankle weights. Lean your hands against the wall and extend one leg back with the toe off the ground.

2. Lift your leg higher without raising your hips.

Perform the movement dynamically 15 times, then pause for 15 seconds. Repeat 3 times with both legs.

Exercise 9

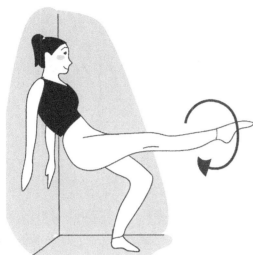

1. Lean your shoulders against the wall and extend one leg in front of you, bending the supporting leg.

2. Slowly perform clockwise, circular movements with your foot 15 times, then pause for 15 seconds. Repeat 3 times with both legs.

Then slowly perform counterclockwise circular movements with your foot 15 times, then pause for 15 seconds. Repeat 3 times with both legs.

Final relaxation

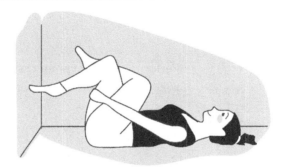

Rest your back on the floor and cross your legs against your chest. Grasp the bottom thigh with your hands.
Exhale slowly with your mouth ajar and relax your face muscles. Repeat for 2 minutes on both sides.

Tip of the Day: Soup for every season

Soup is a meal suitable for more than the winter season; it is a meal that can also be eaten in the spring and summer, with a few tricks. If it is a hot day, soup can be eaten at room temperature, with the addition of fresh flavors reminiscent of summer, such as mint and basil leaves. Also consider making creamed soups instead of the classic vegetable soup, such as leek, potato and carrot. Squash, carrot and celery are velvety soups that are both satisfying and low in calories. In Spain, in the summer it is customary to blend all the seasonal ingredients (tomatoes, cucumbers, celery, onions, garlic) with ice and make a delicious Gazpacho.

Imagination is your ally in the kitchen and friend to your figure!

WORKOUT DAY 24

Exercise 1

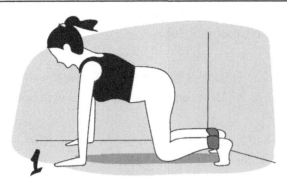 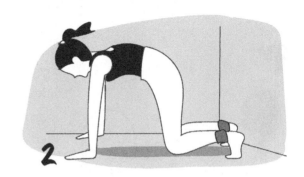

1. Use ankle weights. Rest your hands and knees on the floor, keeping your back flat.

2. Round your back and lift your knees off the floor. Take three long breaths.

Perform the movement slowly 15 times, then pause for 15 seconds. Repeat 3 times.

Exercise 2

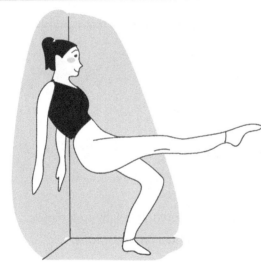

Lean your shoulders against the wall and extend one leg straight front of you, keeping the supporting leg bent. Take 9 long breaths.

Perform the movement slowly 15 times, then pause for 15 seconds. Repeat 3 times with both legs.

Exercise 3

Lean your shoulders against the wall and extend one leg straight in front of you, keeping the supporting leg straight. Take 9 long breaths.

Perform the movement slowly 15 times, then pause for 15 seconds. Repeat 3 times with both legs.

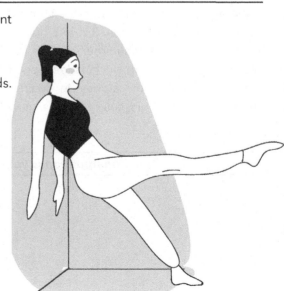

Exercise 4

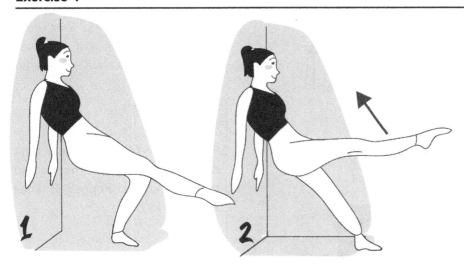

1. Lean your shoulders against the wall and extend one leg in front of you, bending the supporting leg.

2. Lift the leg above horizontal and straighten the supporting leg.

Perform the movement dynamically 15 times, then pause for 15 seconds. Repeat 3 times with both legs.

Exercise 5

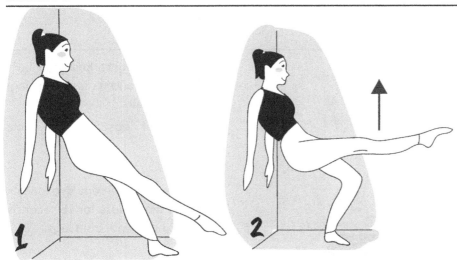

1. Lean your shoulders against the wall and extend one leg in front of you, keeping the supporting leg straight.

2. Lift the leg above horizontal and bend the supporting leg.

Perform the movement dynamically 15 times, then pause for 15 seconds. Repeat 3 times with both legs.

Exercise 6

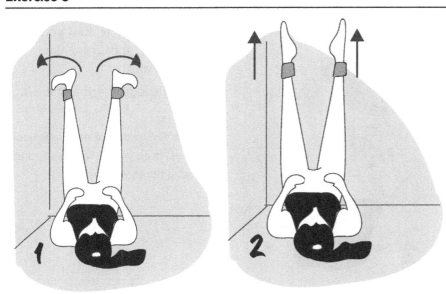

1. Use ankle weights. Rest your back on the floor and put your legs against the wall. Flex your feet and take three long breaths.

2. Point your toes and take three long breaths.

Perform the movement slowly 15 times, then pause for 15 seconds. Repeat 3 times with both legs.

Exercise 7

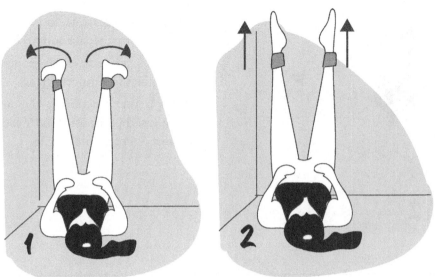

1. Use ankle weights. Rest your back on the floor and put your legs against the wall. Flex your feet.

2. Point your toes.

Perform the movement dynamically 15 times, then pause for 15 seconds. Repeat 3 times with both legs.

Exercise 8

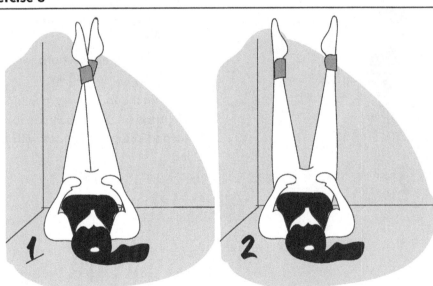

1. Use ankle weights. Rest your back on the floor and cross your legs against the wall.

2. Open your legs and then cross them again.

Perform the movement dynamically 15 times, then pause for 15 seconds. Repeat 3 times with both legs.

Exercise 9

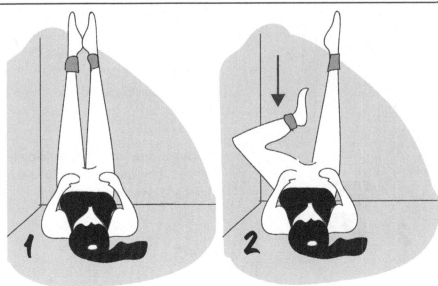

1. Use ankle weights. Rest your back on the floor and cross your legs against the wall.

2. Bend one leg, then straighten it.

Perform the movement dynamically 15 times, then pause for 15 seconds. Repeat 3 times with both legs.

Exercise 10

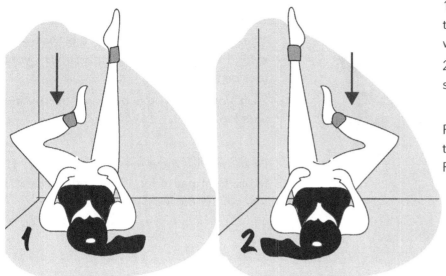

1. Use ankle weights. Rest your back on the floor and put your legs against the wall, bending one leg.

2. Then bend the other leg and then straighten it again.

Perform the movement dynamically 15 times, then pause for 15 seconds. Repeat 3 times with both legs.

Final relaxation

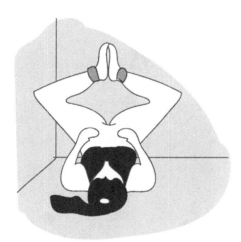

Rest your back on the floor and bend your legs with the soles of your feet together; take deep breaths.

Exhale slowly with your mouth ajar and relax your face muscles. Straighten your legs, then repeat for 2 minutes.

Tip of the Day: What time is best for consuming pasta?

Lunch is a better time than dinner to consume a pasta dish; there are several reasons for this. Pasta is rich in energy-giving carbohydrates and takes a long time to digest. Therefore, at lunch, the body has more time to use the energy and digest the carbohydrates. If you want to keep your weight under control and have peaceful nights without feeling heavy, choose to have carbohydrates only at lunchtime, while choosing protein for dinner.

Paying attention to details improves fitness and your life!

WORKOUT DAY 25

Exercise 1

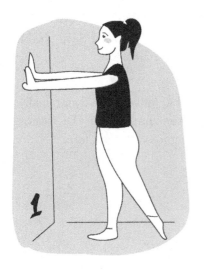 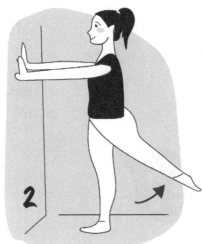

1. Lean your hands against the wall and extend one leg back behind you with your toes on the ground.

2. Lift your leg to the back without raising your hips.

Perform the movement dynamically 15 times, then pause for 15 seconds. Repeat 3 times with both legs.

Exercise 2

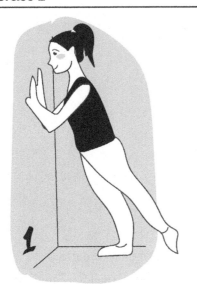 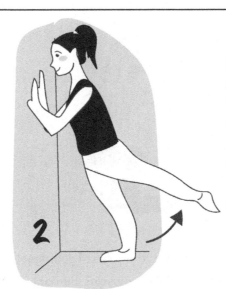

1. Lean your hands against the wall and bend your arms. Extend one leg back with your toes slightly off the ground.

2. Lift your leg without raising your hips.

Perform the movement dynamically 15 times, then pause for 15 seconds. Repeat 3 times with both legs.

Exercise 3

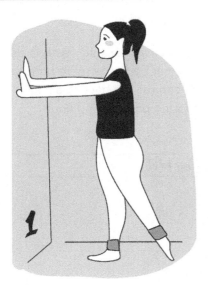 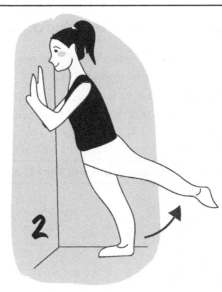

1. Lean your hands against the wall with outstretched arms. Extend one leg behind you, toes slightly off the ground.

2. Bend your arms and lift your leg higher without raising your hips.

Perform the movement dynamically 15 times, then pause for 15 seconds. Repeat 3 times with both legs.

Exercise 4

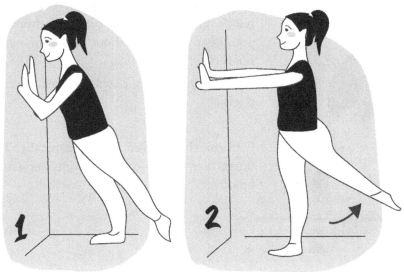

1. Lean your hands against the wall, arms bent. Extend one leg back, toes slightly off the ground.

2. Straighten your arms and lift your leg behind you without raising your hips.

Perform the movement dynamically 15 times, then pause for 15 seconds. Repeat 3 times with both legs.

Exercise 5

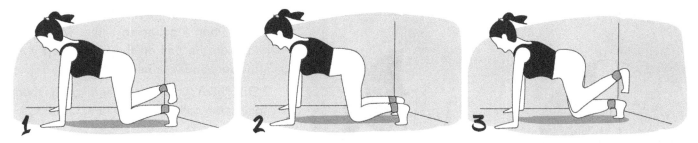

1. Use ankle weights. Rest your hands and knees on the floor, keeping your back flat. Lift one leg off the floor and take three long breaths.

2. Return your leg to the floor.

3. Lift the other leg and take three long breaths.

Perform the movement slowly 15 times, then pause for 15 seconds. Repeat 3 times.

Exercise 6

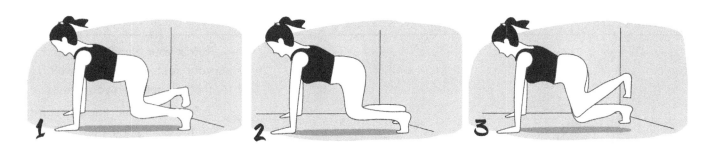

1. Keep your knees lifted off the ground and your hands on the floor, back flat. Lift one leg off the ground and take three long breaths.

2. Return your foot to the ground, without resting your knee.

3. Lift the other foot off the ground and take three long breaths.

Perform the movement slowly 15 times, then pause for 15 seconds. Repeat 3 times.

Exercise 7

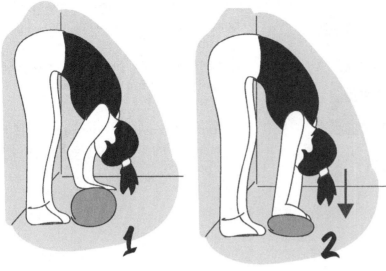

1. Rest your legs against the wall and your hands on the ball on the ground in front of you. Keep your arms bent and your neck relaxed.

2. Extend your arms, pushing them against the ball.

Perform the movement dynamically 15 times, then pause for 15 seconds. Repeat 3 times.

Exercise 8

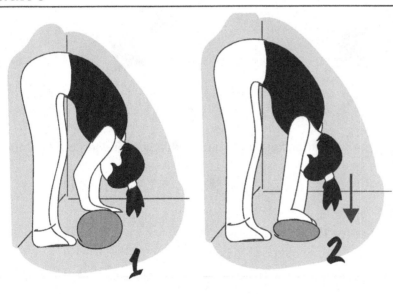

1. Rest your legs against the wall, your hands on the ball on the floor. Keep your arms bent and your neck relaxed.

2. Straighten your arms and push them against the ball. Take three long breaths.

Perform the movement slowly 15 times, then pause for 15 seconds. Repeat 3 times.

Exercise 9

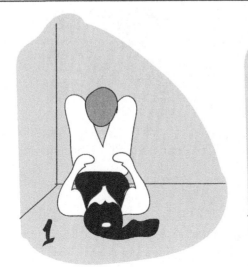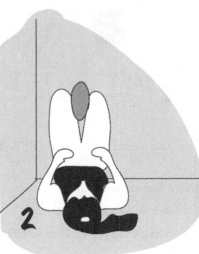

1. Rest your back on the floor with your feet against the wall. Hold the ball between your knees.

2. Squeeze your knees together, compressing the ball. Take three long breaths.

Perform the movement slowly 15 times, then pause for 15 seconds. Repeat 3 times.

Exercise 10

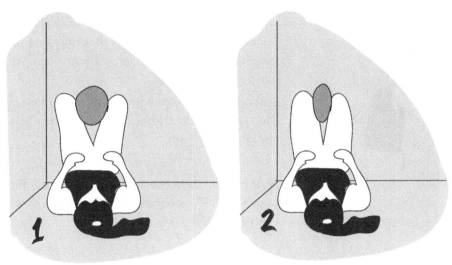

1. Rest your back on the floor and your feet against the wall. Hold the ball between your knees.

2. Squeeze your knees together and compress the ball.

Perform the movement dynamically 15 times, then pause for 15 seconds. Repeat 3 times.

Final relaxation

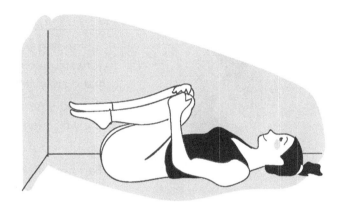

Lying on the floor, bend your knees to your chest and take long breaths for 3 minutes.

Tip of the Day: Do you love yourself enough?

Whatever effort you are making to get back into shape, you will never be satisfied if you do not love yourself first. Your body has a unique and special shape that is unlikely to resemble that of the young women in magazines. Those photos are often retouched by advertising graphic designers, while reality, true beauty, and naturalness are what you see every day around you and in the mirror. Look at yourself and try to love what you see and appreciate your shape. You need to feel good on the inside so that this is also reflected on the outside. Losing weight is fine if it is necessary for your health. But even more important is to understand what your ideal weight is, your ideal shape, and to love yourself as you are.

Having a healthy body and mind is the basis of everything!

WORKOUT DAY 26

Exercise 1

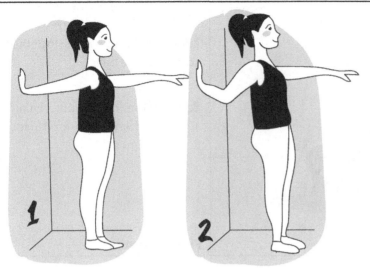

1. Standing in front of the wall, bring one arm forward and one arm behind you. Rest your hand against the wall.

2. Bend your arm, bringing your back closer to the wall. Take three long breaths. Then straighten your arm.

Perform the movement slowly 15 times, then pause for 15 seconds. Repeat 3 times with both arms.

Exercise 2

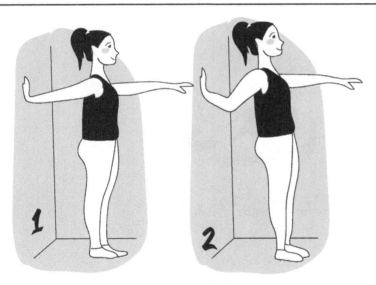

1. Standing in front of the wall, bring one arm forward and one arm behind you. Rest your hand against the wall.

2. Bend your arm, bringing your back closer to the wall, then straighten it.

Perform the movement dynamically 15 times, then pause for 15 seconds. Repeat 3 times with both arms.

Exercise 3

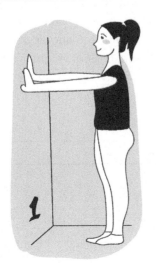 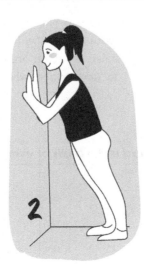

1. Standing in front of the wall, place your hands against the wall.

2. Bend your arms, bringing your upper body closer to the wall. Take three long breaths. Then straighten your arms.

Perform the movement slowly 15 times, then pause for 15 seconds. Repeat 3 times.

Exercise 4

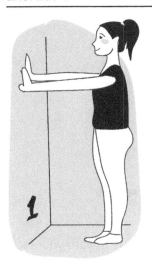 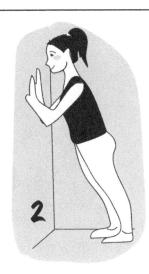

1.Standing in front of the wall, lean your hands against the wall.

2.Bend your arms, bringing your upper body closer to the wall. Then straighten your arms.

Perform the movement dynamically 15 times, then pause for 15 seconds. Repeat 3 times.

Exercise 5

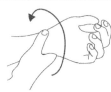

Pause and loosen both wrists before continuing.

Rotate your wrists in a twisting motion to the right and left.

Perform a gentle massage.

Exercise 6

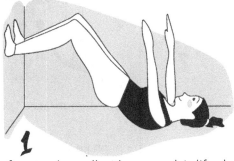 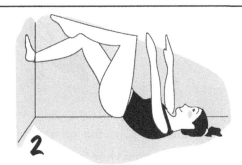

1. Place your feet on the wall with your pelvis lifted off the ground. Stretch your arms towards the ceiling.

2. Bring one leg towards you and take three long breaths. Keep your gaze upward.

Perform the movement slowly 15 times, then pause for 15 seconds. Repeat 3 times with both legs.

Exercise 7

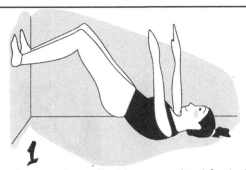 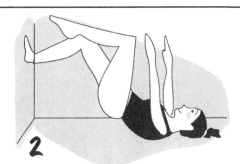

1. Place your feet on the wall with your pelvis lifted off the ground. Stretch your arms towards the ceiling.

2. Bend one leg then place your foot back on the wall.

Perform the movement dynamically 15 times, then pause for 15 seconds. Repeat 3 times with both legs.

Exercise 8

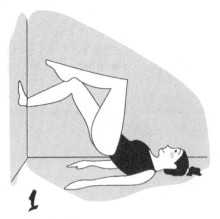 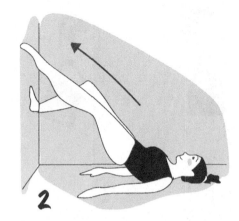

1. Keeping your feet firm against the wall, go into the bridge position. Exhale and bring one knee toward your face.

2. Inhale and extend the leg towards the wall.

Perform the movement dynamically 15 times, then pause for 15 seconds. Repeat 3 times, then switch legs.

Exercise 9

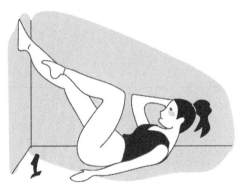 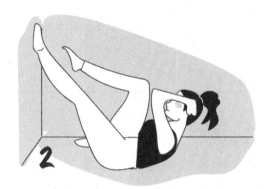

1. Keeping one foot firmly against the wall, exhale and bring your other knee toward your face. Take three long breaths, then inhale and place the leg back on the wall.

2. Exhale and bring the other knee toward your face. Take three long breaths, then inhale and extend the leg back to the wall.

Perform the movement slowly 15 times, then pause for 15 seconds. Repeat 3 times.

Exercise 9

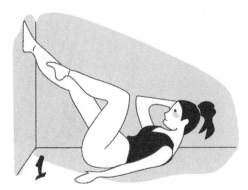 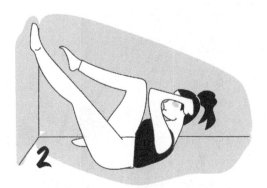

1. Keeping one foot firmly against the wall, bring your knee toward your face, then extend your leg.

2. Bring the other knee toward your face, then extend the leg.

Perform the movement dynamically 15 times, then pause for 15 seconds. Repeat 3 times.

Exercise 10

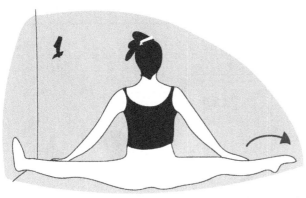 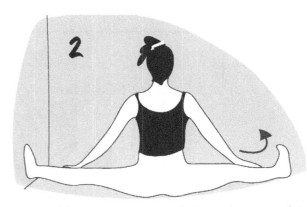

1. Keeping one foot firmly against the wall, spread your legs wide and keep your torso still. Point the toes of the free foot toward the floor.
2. Then flex your foot so the toes face upward.

Perform the movement dynamically 15 times, then pause for 15 seconds. Repeat 3 times with both legs.

Final relaxation

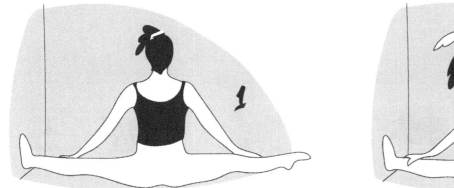 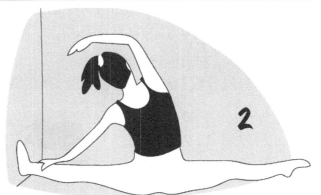

1. Keeping one foot firmly against the wall, spread your legs and keep your torso still.
2. Extend the arm that's away from the wall over your head and bend toward the wall. Take long breaths.

Perform the movement slowly 15 times, then pause for 15 seconds. Repeat 3 times on both sides.

Tip of the Day: The importance of relationships

Remember that this challenge you have taken on is not just about weight loss. It's about taking care of yourself, and no one should distract you from your wellness goals. So now is the time to choose who in your circle of acquaintances can truly support you versus those who are not supportive.

Seek support from those who make you feel good; the warmth of a hug and the pleasure of laughing with a loved one are important emotional boosters.

The quality of your life also depends on the quality of your relationships.

WORKOUT DAY 27

Exercise 1

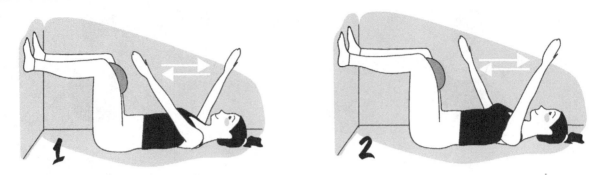

1. With your feet placed firmly on the wall, hold the ball between your knees. Bring your outstretched arms up at an angle, with your shoulders resting firmly on the floor.

2. Energetically alternate your arms forward and backward.

Perform the dynamic movement 15 times, then pause for 15 seconds. Repeat 3 times.

Exercise 2

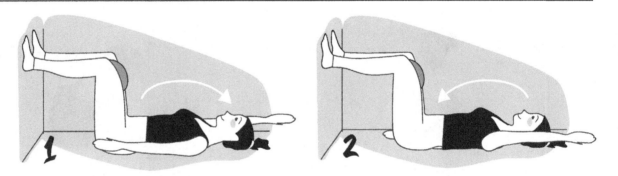

1. With your feet placed firmly on the wall, hold the ball between your knees. Exhale and reach one arm straight overhead and one down at your side; contract your abs.

2. Inhale and alternate arm positions slowly, following the breath.

Perform the movement following the breath 15 times, then pause for 15 seconds. Repeat 3 times.

Exercise 3

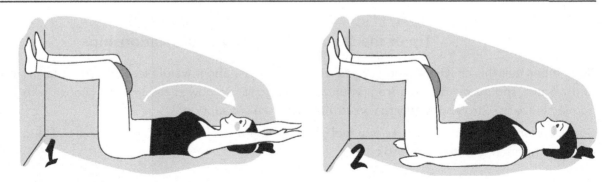

1. With your feet placed firmly on the wall, hold the ball between your knees. Inhale and stretch your arms stretched over your head; contract your abs.

2. Exhale and bring your arms up to the ceiling to rest at your sides, slowly, following the breath.

Perform the movement following the breath 15 times, then pause for 15 seconds. Repeat 3 times.

Exercise 4

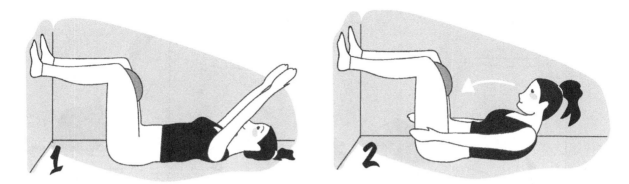

1. With your feet placed firmly on the wall, hold the ball between your knees and reach your arms at an angle over your head.
2. Bring your arms outstretched forward and lift your shoulders off the floor. Contract your abs and take 3 long breaths.

Perform the movement following the breath 15 times, then pause for 15 seconds. Repeat 3 times.

Exercise 5

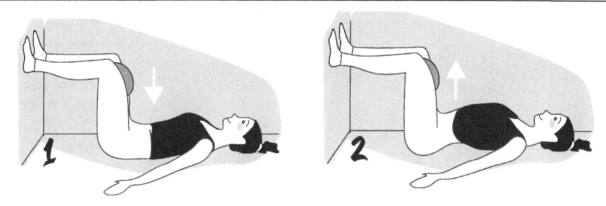

1. Keep your feet firm against the wall, your arms along your sides, and the ball between your knees. Take a long breath and rest all vertebrae on the floor.
2. Take another long breath and lift your chest off the floor.

Perform the movement following the breath 15 times, then pause for 15 seconds. Repeat 3 times.

Exercise 6

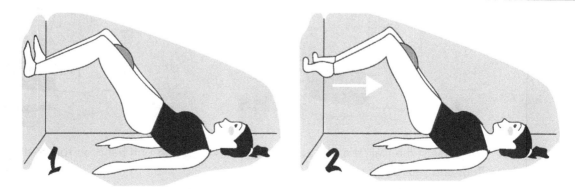

1. Lie with your feet on the wall and the ball between your knees. Get into the bridge position. Keep your arms along your sides.
2. Lift your heels and contract your glutes. Take three long breaths.

Perform the movement slowly 15 times, then pause for 15 seconds. Repeat 3 times.

Exercise 7

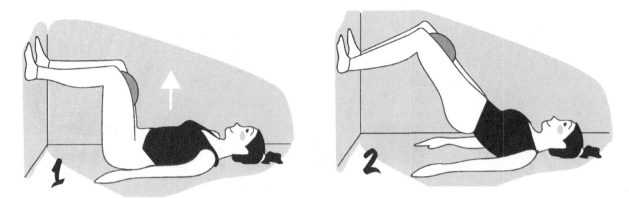

1. Lie with your feet on the wall and the ball between your knees.

2. Get into the bridge position with your arms along your sides. Contract your glutes and take three long breaths.

Perform the movement slowly 15 times, then pause for 15 seconds. Repeat 3 times.

Exercise 8

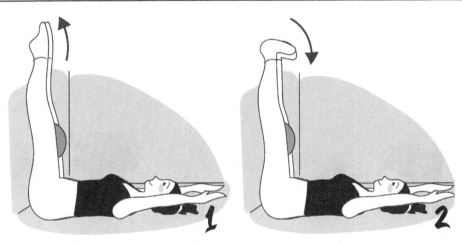

1. Rest your outstretched legs against the wall, your back flat on the floor. Hold the ball between your knees. Point your toes toward the ceiling.

2. Then flex your feet so your toes face the wall behind you.

Perform the movement dynamically 15 times, then pause for 15 seconds. Repeat 3 times.

Exercise 9

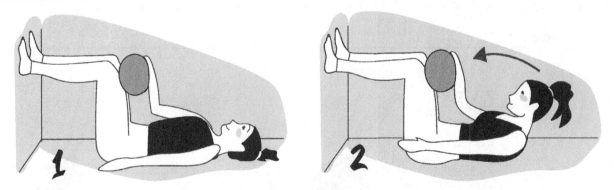

1. Keep your feet firm against the wall, the ball resting on your knees and one hand on top of the ball. Keep your back flat on the floor and your other arm at your side.

2. Lift your shoulders off the floor. Press your hand against the ball and take 3 long breaths.

Perform the movement following the breath 15 times, then pause for 15 seconds. Repeat 3 times with both arms.

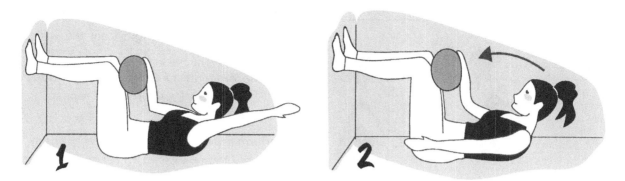

1. Keep your feet firm against the wall, the ball resting on your knees and one hand on top of the ball. Lift your shoulders off the ground and bring your other arm over your head.

2. Press your hand against the ball and bring your other arm along your side.

Perform the movement dynamically 15 times, then pause for 15 seconds. Repeat 3 times with both arms.

Final relaxation

Lunge forward on one leg with the other bent and resting against the wall. Keep your hands on the floor and look forward.

Raise and lower your pelvis 15 times. Then take a 15-second break. Repeat 3 times.

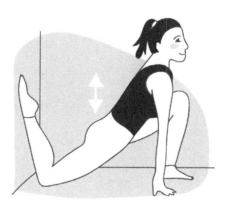

Tip of the Day: The shopping list

Achieving your goals is easier when you feel gratified by foods that are healthy but tasty at the same time. One of the best ways to achieve this is to make a list of the foods you like and look for the best possible healthy alternative that satisfies your tastes. You can, for example, substitute French fries for golden baked potatoes, and you can substitute cookies for whole wheat bread with honey. Making a wish list allows you to then compile a varied shopping list full of healthy foods so that you can maintain control over your daily diet without losing your good mood.

A satisfactory meal is a strong incentive for goal achievement.

WORKOUT DAY 28

Exercise 1

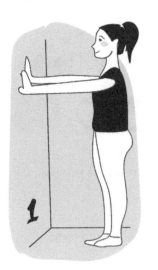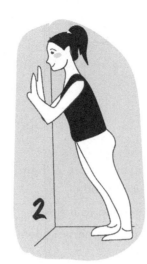

1.Standing at arms' length from the wall, lean on your hands.

2.Bend your arms to bring your upper body closer to the wall. Then extend your arms and repeat.

Perform the movement dynamically (briskly, with energy) 15 times, then pause for 15 seconds. Repeat 3 times.

Exercise 2

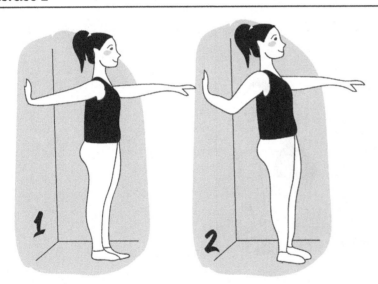

1.Standing in front of the wall, bring one arm forward and one arm behind you. Rest the hand behind you against the wall.

2.Bend your arm to bring your back closer to the wall. Then extend the arm and repeat.

Perform the movement dynamically 15 times, then pause for 15 seconds. Repeat 3 times with both arms.

Exercise 3

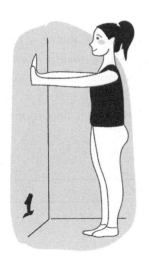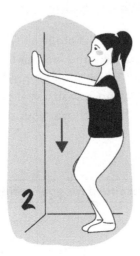

1.Standing in front of the wall, place your hands on the wall.

2.Without moving your arms, bend your knees and lower your body straight down. Then straighten your legs and repeat.

Perform the movement dynamically 15 times, then pause for 15 seconds. Repeat 3 times.

Exercise 4

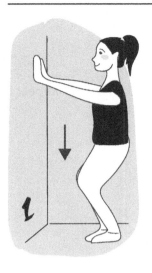 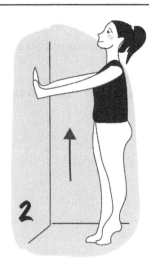

1. Standing in front of the wall with feet close together, place your hands on the wall.

2. Lift your heels off the ground without moving your arms. Then lower your heels to the ground.

Perform the movement dynamically 15 times, then pause for 15 seconds. Repeat 3 times.

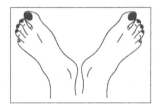

Exercise 5

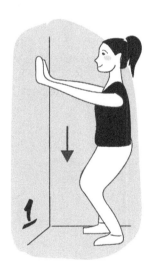 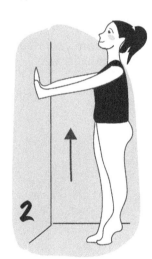

1. Standing in front of the wall with your feet hip-width apart, place your hands on the wall. Without moving your arms, bend your knees to lower your body.

2. Straighten your legs and lift your heels off the floor, again without moving your arms. Then return to the standing position.

Perform the movement dynamically 15 times, then pause for 15 seconds. Repeat 3 times.

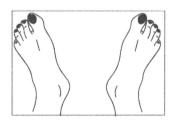

Exercise 6

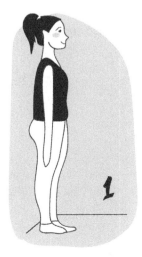 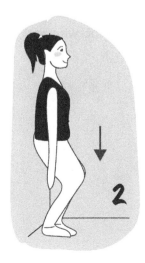

1. Standing in front of the wall, place your hands against the wall. Keep your heels together, toes facing out.

2. Bend your knees to lower your body without moving your back away from the wall. Then stand up straight.

Perform the movement dynamically 15 times, then pause for 15 seconds. Repeat 3 times.

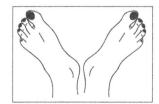

Exercise 7

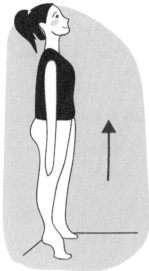

1. Stand in front of the wall with your feet hip-width apart, toes facing out.
2. Rise up onto your toes and then return your heels to the floor.

Perform the movement dynamically 15 times, then pause for 15 seconds. Repeat 3 times.

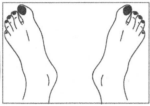

Exercise 8

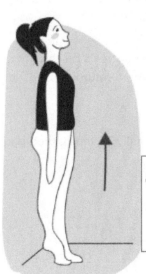

1. Stand with your heels together, toes facing out.
2. Rise up onto your toes and then return your heels to the floor.

Perform the movement slowly 15 times, then pause for 15 seconds. Repeat 3 times.

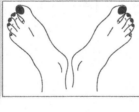

Exercise 8

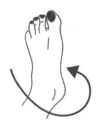

Rotate your ankles clockwise and counterclockwise to loosen the joint.

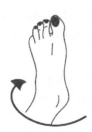

Exercise 9

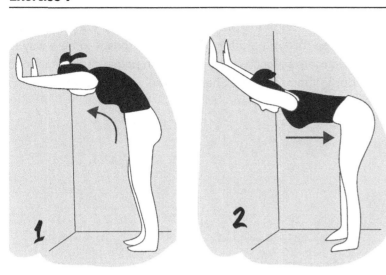

1. Place your hands against the wall, the push against it, hunching your back.

2. Bring your back to a horizontal position.

Perform the movement dynamically 15 times, then pause for 15 seconds. Repeat 3 times.

Exercise 10

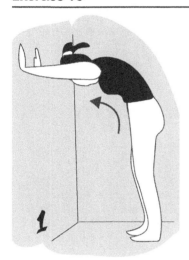 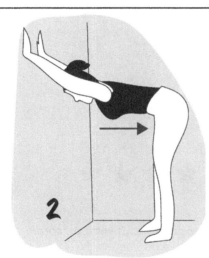

1. Place your hands against the wall and push against it, hunching your back. Hold the position for three long breaths.

2. Bring your back to a horizontal position and take three long breaths.

Perform the movement slowly 15 times, then pause for 15 seconds. Repeat 3 times.

Tip of the Day: Gratification

You have completed your first workout: Congratulations! To get the results you set for yourself, you just need to keep your focus on your goals and never neglect your emotional well-being. Be kind to yourself and proud of the journey you have embarked on by giving yourself a reward of gratification such as a hot shower, a phone call with a friend, or watching a good movie.

Remember that you are extraordinary, regardless of the number on the scale.

Conclusion

Congratulations, you have come to the end of this challenge. Through the practice of Wall Pilates, I discovered an inner strength that goes beyond my physical form, and I hope that you did too. This book is meant to be a way to find the tools that unite the body and mind so that you have more balance in daily life. Each page is an invitation to transform, be aware of, and have gratitude toward your body. I hope this book has inspired you to value the beauty and strength within you, leading you to live in harmony with yourself.

Your support means a lot to me and would be invaluable in spreading my work.

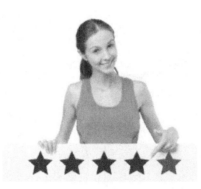

https://wallpilatestotalbody.flyedition.com/

If you enjoyed this book, please leave a review!

MORE BOOKS BY THIS AUTHOR ARE AVAILABLE ON AMAZON

Made in the USA
Las Vegas, NV
11 January 2024

84202917R00063